PROFESSOR R. W. FOGEL
HARVARD UNIVERSITY
1737 CAMBRIDGE ST., RM. G-7
CAMBRIDGE, MA. 02138

6/1/78

THE MAKING OF THE MODERN BRITISH DIET

The Making of the Modern British Diet

Edited by
DEREK ODDY *and* DEREK MILLER

CROOM HELM LONDON

ROWMAN AND LITTLEFIELD TOTOWA N.J.

© 1976 D.J. Oddy and D.S. Miller

Croom Helm Ltd 2-10 St. John's Road SW11

ISBN 0-85664-252-5

First published in the United States 1976 by
Rowman and Littlefield
81 Adams Drive
TOTOWA, New Jersey.

ISBN 0-87471-803-1

Printed in Great Britain by Biddles of Guildford

CONTENTS

1. Editors' Introduction — 7

Part One: The Supply of Food

2. Nutrition, technology and the growth of the British biscuit industry, 1820-1900 — 13
   T.A.B. Corley
3. The 'consumer revolution' and the growth of factory foods: changing patterns of bread and cereal-eating in Britain in the twentieth century — 26
   E.J.T. Collins
4. The development of the meat industry — 44
   E.F. Williams
5. The growth of the sugar trade and refining industry — 58
   G.N. Johnstone
6. The London milk trade, 1900-1930 — 65
   E.H. Whetham
7. The cocoa and chocolate industry in the nineteenth century — 77
   J. Othick
8. The British tea trade in the nineteenth century — 91
   P. Mathias

Part Two: Factors Influencing Consumption

9. The agricultural labourer's standard of living in Kent, 1790-1840 — 103
   T.L. Richardson
10. Drink and working-class living standards in Britain, 1870-1914 — 117
    A.E. Dingle
11. Regional variations in food habits — 135
    D.E. Allen
12. The corner shop: the development of the grocery and general provisions trade — 148
    J.M. Blackman
13. J. Lyons and Co. Ltd: caterers and food manufacturers, 1894-1939 — 161
    D.J. Richardson
14. The development of the food-canning industry in Britain during the inter-war period — 173
    J.P. Johnston

Part Three: A Nutritional Evaluation

15. Developments leading to present-day nutritional knowledge 189
    D.F. Hollingsworth
16. Some basic principles of nutrition 196
    J. Yudkin
17. Nutrition surveys 202
    D.S. Miller
18. A nutritional analysis of historical evidence: the working-class diet, 1880-1914 214
    D.J. Oddy

Index 232

CONTRIBUTORS

Mr. D.E. Allen, formerly a market research executive, and now on the staff of the Social Science Research Council, but writes in his private capacity.

Dr. Janet M. Blackman, Lecturer in Economic and Social History, University of Hull.

Dr. E.J.T. Collins, Associate Director, Institute of Agricultural History, University of Reading.

Mr. T.A.B. Corley, Senior Lecturer in Economics, University of Reading.

Mr. A.E. Dingle, Lecturer in Economic History, Monash University, Australia.

Miss Dorothy F. Hollingsworth, Director, British Nutrition Foundation.

Mr. J.P. Johnston, Research Economic Historian, University of Bristol.

Mr. G.N. Johnstone, Chief Press Officer, John Laing and Co. Ltd., and formerly of Tate and Lyle Ltd.

Prof. P. Mathias, Chichele Professor of Economic History, All Souls College, University of Oxford.

Mr. D.S. Miller, Research Nutritionist, Queen Elizabeth College, University of London.

Dr. D.J. Oddy, Senior Lecturer in Economic History, Ealing Technical College.

Mr. J. Othick, Lecturer in Economic History, The Queen's University, Belfast.

Dr. D.J. Richardson, Assistant Master, Rugby School.

Mr. T. L. Richardson, Lecturer in Economic History, University of Kent.

Miss Edith H. Whetham, Fellow of Newnham College and formerly Gilbey Lecturer in the History and Economics of Agriculture, University of Cambridge.

Prof. E.F. Williams, formerly of J. Sainsbury Ltd.

Prof. J. Yudkin, Emeritus Professor of Nutrition and Dietetics, Queen Elizabeth College, University of London.

1 INTRODUCTION

D.J. ODDY and D.S. MILLER

Food is the physiological basis of man's existence; without it his being is limited in time and the survival of his species an impossibility. But food has also greater significance in society than its physiological function. It is essentially an expression of a society's culture and may play many roles other than physiological in terms of both personal and group relationships. Food is one of the basic sensual pleasures in human life and, as such, forms a major element in the socialisation of the child, in expressions of love and courtship, in the establishment of a gift relationship, and may even serve to express social disapproval. One complexity in any discussion of food is that not everything edible is food: 'A food has no meaning if a man does not give it a meaning by willingly eating it.'[1] Thus forms of preparation, cooking and serving food become ritualised[2] and even, in some cases, develop into techniques to allow man to persist in eating foods such as maize and some crustaceans which otherwise would be harmful to his health.

The importance given to food by a society has shown a remarkable variation during man's history. In the ancient world, the sacrifice of animals and certain foodstuffs was an essential part of public ceremony and religious practice. Undoubtedly, the highest emanations of ancient philosophy were related to the eating of meals — the last days of Socrates, Plato's symposium, Christ's last supper. By contrast, some societies have selected foodstuffs to apply some of the strictest taboos by which man has regulated the behaviour of his group.[3] Yet, to quote Dr. Magnus Pyke: 'The dogma of the west, which it is heresy to challenge, is that our dietary habits are based on reason: it is only remote foreign tribes which believe in taboos.'[4] Nevertheless, the reader will recognise that aversion to eating the flesh of horses, dogs, rats, or spiders, which exists in all western industrialised societies, is in fact a taboo and, with the possible exception of horseflesh, one for which no rational explanation has been advanced.[5] One might even decline food habits as: I have preferences, you have prejudices, he is a crank. Our purpose in this book, however, is less concerned with a general understanding of the pyscho-social aspects of food than with the specific question of the role of food during industrialisation and urbanisation in Britain.

In Britain, the first country to undergo this process of modernisation, there were profound changes in British society and yet the role of food has attracted little academic interest. Until recently, the lack of studies of food have been almost a gap in the conceptual framework of economic history. Some studies, such as Sir William Ashley's *The Bread of our Forefathers,* are notable exceptions, but seminal works such as *The Englishman's Food*[6] and *The History and Social Influence of the Potato*[7] have come from the pens of practising scientists rather than historians.

In a book formed from a collection of research papers which reflect the diversity of their authors' interests, we must emphasise the overall coherence of the papers which we have brought together. Part One of the book contains a series of commodity studies covering bread, cereals, biscuits, meat, milk, tea and cocoa which reflect trends in the supply of some of the foods in the British diet during the nineteenth and early twentieth centuries. This is by no means a comprehensive list of the commodities entering the shops and markets nor does it reflect a particular order of importance. In some respects, indeed, it leaves gaps which the reader may find frustrating, partly because studies dealing with the supply of food need to be seen in conjunction with some broad assessment of consumption patterns and partly because some foods are omitted. One of the most interesting commodity groups, for example, is that of vegetables for which the changing basis of supply to the newly urbanised areas has not been adequately researched, despite the general interest in agriculture in the later nineteenth century. These studies form a traditional approach within economic history to the functions of production and trade. All, in fact, refer to changes in demand for foods but we have separated them from the group of papers in Part Two in which the emphasis is predominantly on consumption, either through the study of living standards or consumer preference or through the presentation of food and the organisation of its outlets to the consumer. The final part of the book contains an approach which is undoubtedly new for an historical work. Until now, historians have either lacked sufficient basic nutritional knowledge on which to base even qualitative assessments (was there, for instance, as Peter Laslett implies, pellagra in seventeenth-century England?)[8] or have not been presented with the possibilities offered by nutritional techniques to evaluate historical evidence.

We hope that historians may find not only some basic nutrition but also some guidance to the pitfalls and possibilities that are opened up. A study of how nutritional knowledge developed may make historians aware of the difficulties of using contemporary evidence in the late nineteenth or early twentieth centuries, when comments offered on diet may not be accepted as valid in the light of modern nutritional knowledge. The two final papers contributed by ourselves are concerned on the one hand with the difficulties of carrying out dietary surveys and on the other with the possibilities which are available to the historian to make a quantitative evaluation of historical evidence utilising modern nutritional knowledge combined with the facilities offered by computer techniques. These final papers may raise questions in readers' minds regarding the validity and utility of applying these techniques to historical data. It is reasonable to ask how accurate nutritional analysis can be when based on historical evidence. Certainly we do not expect research workers to adopt quantitative techniques because it is fashionable to do so. Some care is needed, clearly, in the analysis of historical data in view of the usual lack of information about methods of food preservation and cooking, and uncertainty about quality. It is true that this may throw some doubt on the values calculated for vitamins, but it can hardly invalidate the protein and energy values of the diet. In any case, if the same techniques are used to compare diets of different origins, the relative nutrient contents are meaningful and there is an obvious advantage in making quantitative comparisons of otherwise descriptive material. The fear that historical analysis is insufficiently accurate should be tempered by the discussion of current problems of carrying out dietary surveys. The parallel which is drawn in this paper between problems of economic development viewed historically and those of the Third World today should encourage research into areas of British history which have relevance in terms of general economic development.

These papers have not come together either by chance or by conscious design: in either case the balance and scope might have been different. The contributions to this book are papers which have been read to a research seminar in the Department of Nutrition at Queen Elizabeth College. The seminar is a multi-disciplinary group containing historians, nutritionists and food scientists and owes much for its original inspiration to Professor John Yudkin as former head of department, and to the breadth of interests which the department has always contained. From 1962, when John McKenzie began work in social nutrition at Queen Elizabeth College, historical studies have formed an important part of the programme. Much enthusiasm and unflagging support for the work has come from Theo Barker, Professor of Economic and Social History at the University of Kent, and Stewart Truswell, Professor of Nutrition and current Head of the Department of Nutrition at Queen Elizabeth College has sought to maintain and encourage the activities of the seminar. The value of this work was brought out by symposia held at Queen Elizabeth College which combined both academic interests and those of marketing and industry. Its interdisciplinary nature can best be seen in *Changing Food Habits*[9] and a more specifically historical work came later with *Our Changing Fare*.[10] Even so, both works are now out of print and may not be either readily available or well-known to many social scientists today.

We hope that this volume will prove a worthy successor to the earlier works and, in particular, that it will highlight growing research interests into food history and encourage further studies of this aspect of economic development in Britain.

Notes

1. J. Tremolières, 'A behavioural approach to organoleptic properties of food', *Proceedings of the Nutrition Society*, Vol. 29, 2 (1970), p.286.
2. See C. Levi-Strauss, 'The culinary triangle', *New Society*, 22 December 1966, for this approach.
3. See Tremolières, op. cit., for a discussion of food as part of the *volupté* of Latin civilisation.
4. M. Pyke, 'Man eats dog', *The Listener*, 16 March 1967.
5. Pyke, op. cit., suggests that Pope Gregory III ordered Boniface to forbid horse-flesh to the converted German tribes.
6. J.C. Drummond and A. Wilbraham, *The Englishman's Food*, revised edition, edited by D. Hollingsworth, Cape, 1957.
7. R.N. Salaman, *The History and Social Influence of the Potato*, Cambridge University Press, 1949.
8. P. Laslett, *The World we have Lost*, Methuen, 1971, p.123.
9. J. Yudkin and J.C. McKenzie (eds.), *Changing Food Habits*, MacGibbon and Kee, 1964.
10. T.C. Barker, J.C. McKenzie, and J. Yudkin (eds.), *Our Changing Fare*, MacGibbon and Kee, 1966.

ACKNOWLEDGEMENTS

We are grateful to the Institute of Agricultural History, University of Reading, for permission to reprint Miss Edith Whetham's paper, 'The London Milk Trade 1900–1930', and also to the Editors of the *Economic History Review* for permission to reprint Mr. A.E. Dingle's paper, 'Drink and Working-Class Living Standards in Britain, 1870–1914'. The paper by Professor John Yudkin, 'Some Basic Principles of Nutrition', is adapted from *This Nutrition Business* to be published by Davis Poynter.

PART ONE: THE SUPPLY OF FOOD

2 NUTRITION, TECHNOLOGY AND THE GROWTH OF THE BRITISH BISCUIT INDUSTRY 1820–1900[1]

T.A.B. CORLEY

The popularity of the fancy biscuit is enormous. In 1972 the industry's sales were valued at no less than £208 millions.[2] The object of this paper is therefore to put forward some reasons for the growth of what is now such a flourishing industry. To the economist, the biscuit is an ideal example of a consumer's good that is moderately inexpensive and available in many different varieties. Yet few among his number, or his associates the economic historians, have done much systematic work on the development of this or other industries, in the sense of tracing exactly how groups of firms came to be linked up in the kinds of industrial groupings we are familiar with today. The present paper is offered as a case study of a typical medium-sized industry during its formative years.

In brief, a combination of changes in people's nutritional habits on one side and in technology on the other side created the conditions for the biscuit industry to emerge as it did. That these conditions were translated into reality was the achievement of some able entrepreneurs who saw the technical and marketing opportunities and pressed them to the point of a break-through between the 1820s and 1850s. In fact there were two quite separate developments, in ship's biscuits as well as in the fancy kind.

Ship's Biscuits

The biscuit as we know it here is essentially a British invention and differs from the American cracker or its softer and more cake-like counterpart in Europe. Its crispness, at least in the plain and semi-sweet varieties, probably owes much to the ship's biscuit which in our maritime nation has been produced for many centuries before fancy biscuits appeared on the market. Shakespeare knew very well its unappetising nature when he used the simile 'as dry as the remainder biscuit after a voyage'. If, as some biographers have suggested, he went to sea as a very young man, he could well have purchased this kind of biscuit from the small bakeries situated near the wharves where vessels docked. A few such bakeries survived until within living memory, the baker and an assistant usually being enough to carry out the various tasks from kneading the dough to rolling, shaping and cutting the biscuits by hand, before baking them in the oven.

Then in the eighteenth century the victualling authorities in the king's dockyards of Deptford, Portsmouth and Plymouth began to set up their own baking establishments for the Royal Navy's needs. Their intention may have been to secure the economies of large-scale production that could not be realised in the small bakeries. At the same time, however, the sequence of wars in that century made it almost impossible to ensure an adequate supply of biscuits since the demand rose very sharply in wartime and then fell back just as drastically once peace returned. By their extensive organisation these establishments achieved a division of labour even more remarkable than the one described in Adam Smith's celebrated pin factory.[3]

The production process really involved creating a human assembly line that economised each workman's movements to the utmost. It was thus highly labour-intensive, the equipment comprising little more than the mixing troughs, a rolling pin and a tool for perforating or 'docking' the uncooked biscuits so as to prevent them from swelling up while being baked. The kneading of the flour and water into dough was carried out manually, for the 'idleman' energetically kneaded by hand for half an hour and then jumped into the trough and trod it with his bare feet. The 'brakeman' had his roller, or brake staff, attached to the wall by a leather thong and sat astride the other end to exert the maximum weight on it, and shuffled to and fro in what was described as a rapid jumping and most uncouth motion over the dough. It was transferred to a moulding board, a table near the oven's mouth. There the 'moulder' cut the dough into slips and then into squares which he moulded into round shapes with his hands. He then laid the shapes on one another two by two and pierced them with the docking instrument mentioned above. When six or eight pairs were ready he threw them on to another table alongside the next workers, the 'furner' and 'pitcher'.

These two by their joint efforts achieved an equally noteworthy expenditure of human strength and agility. The one held a peel or long shovel just inside the oven and the other took from an assistant each biscuit, now once more separated into single pieces, and threw them on to the peel. This the furner agitated so as to arrange them all over the oven floor, the pitcher not taking his eyes off for a second. When the oven was full the door would be closed for about ten minutes. Although the pitcher could throw at the rate of a hundred a minute, it took nearly 600 to fill the oven, and therefore some were baked more thoroughly than others. Moreover, the limits of what could be achieved by existing technology had been reached at a time when extra supplies were urgently needed. Although dockyard production was supplemented by the services of contractors, so grave did the shortage of biscuits become towards the end of the Napoleonic Wars that waggon-loads had to be unpacked in the streets of dockyard towns and taken straight on board warships under sailing orders instead of going through the victualling yards first.

Not until 1833 did the much-needed technological revolution occur, when (Sir) Thomas Grant, superintendent of the Victualling Office at Portsmouth, invented some steam machinery to power certain of these processes. Being technically untrained he was helped by the civil engineer Sir John Rennie, and concentrated on mixing, rolling and cutting. For the mixing process an enormous drum, about 5 feet long and 3 feet in diameter, was used; this contained 18 blades which revolved round a central shaft. As to the raw materials, flour was weighed out in a storeroom above and then shot down by chute into the drum, while the required amount of water was drawn off from a small cistern attached to its top. After two minutes of mixing the dough could be removed through a trap door. It was laid on a board that rested on a nearby table and was reduced in two processes by rollers that weighed 15 cwt. each and were driven by a two-throw crankshaft by means of a connecting rod and a pendulum. The rollers passed backwards and forwards for about three minutes over the dough, which was then cut into smaller pieces and placed under another set of rollers which reduced it to the required thickness. The next process involved pushing the dough under a cutting-out machine, which stamped the dough into hexagonal shapes but without perforating it right through, so that the whole piece could be lifted bodily on to an iron plate. That plate had a handle attached to it for carrying it to the oven. There were nine ovens in all, each heated from a central furnace. Once baked, the biscuits were broken into individual hexagons which thus avoided any waste.

Although no more than partly mechanised, the technical ingenuity of this process can be well appreciated, and the savings in costs were noteworthy. Previously 45 men had been needed to produce about 1,500 lbs. of biscuits an hour, at a direct cost of 1s.6d. (7½p) per cwt., but the new system allowed 16 men and boys to produce almost a ton an hour, or about 50 per cent more, at a cost of 5d. (2p) per cwt., although the expenses of amortising the machinery should be added to that. Moreover, the biscuits were greatly improved in quality, as both the dough mixing and the baking were much more uniform. Interestingly enough, bread baking was not successfully mechanised until nearly the end of the nineteenth century, in Britain at least; there, in contrast with biscuits, the financial benefits have been outweighed by a distinct reduction in palatability.[4]

Fancy Biscuits

While the exact relationship between the technology of ship's biscuits and that of fancy biscuits is not clear, the main facts about the former's mechanisation, with copious illustrations, were available in some detail from various sources by the mid-1830s. These included the *Transactions of the Society of Arts* and Peter Barlow's *Encyclopaedia of Manufactures,* and were later taken up by popular journals such as the

Penny Magazine. Such publications were the kinds available in Mechanics Institutes which the next generation of entrepreneurs patronised.

Biscuits were not originally an article of pleasurable consumption but a medicinal good, much as the charcoal or slimming biscuit is today. The earliest proprietary biscuits were probably the Bath Oliver and Abernethy varieties, invented by Dr. William Oliver (1695-1764) and Dr. John Abernethy (1764-1831) respectively. It was Lemann's of Threadneedle Street, London, founded in 1747 and the doyen of quality biscuit bakers, which brought out the first recorded non-medicinal brand, the York biscuit, to commemorate the marriage of Frederick Duke of York in 1791. All fancy biscuits were made by hand, but some bakeries had a mixing machine turned by a handle. Biscuit bakers tended to operate on a small scale, as pastrycooks or confectioners. Some London firms, on the other hand, made biscuits during the day with the same ovens in which bread had been baked throughout the night.

Both known pioneers of fancy biscuit mechanisation were Quakers: a significant fact not only because Quaker businessmen were proud of dealing in goods that did no harm to anyone, but also because they believed in selling good-quality products, free from adulteration and fairly priced. Thus they set their faces against the kind of deplorable working conditions to be found in many London bakeries of the day. The first of these pioneers was Jonathan Dodgson Carr, a miller and baker of Carlisle who, in the late 1830s, designed some machinery for cutting out and stamping biscuits. Once again he was no engineer, but he received some help from one of the Scott family which ran the printing firm Hudson Scott & Sons of Carlisle. Not surprisingly, therefore, the basic design of this machine was evolved from a hand-operated fly-press. A sheet of kneaded dough was placed on a sliding cloth-covered plate: the cloth allowed the biscuits to be picked up easily. A lever wound the table under hinged cutters, which closed up at the same time and cut out the biscuits into oblong shapes. They were then arranged in a tray to be baked.[5] His firm also had some machinery for kneading, rolling and cutting out, the last-named having a cylindrical cutter for the only other variety he made at that time, a round biscuit. The precise characteristics of the machinery are obscure, but by 1846 it was helping to produce no less than 400 tons of biscuits a year. At least one London biscuit baker at that time was advertising his wares as being manufactured by steam machinery, but the scale of his output is known to have been small.

Naturally enough, Carr's of Carlisle has ever since made much of its invention, claiming that here were the origins of what evolved into a steady process of mechanisation. That claim was disputed by the last of the pioneers to be considered, George Palmer.[6] He was a Quaker who learned his trade as a miller and confectioner, and had more than a layman's interest in engineering matters. In 1841 he joined up with his cousin Thomas Huntley, who made biscuits entirely by hand in his Reading shop, the only mechanical aids being a manually worked brake for the dough. George Palmer immediately had a small steam engine installed in a building behind the shop, no doubt to help with the dough mixing, and by mid-1846 the Huntley & Palmer partnership had nearly £850 worth of machinery and fixtures there, which was successful in more than doubling output between 1841-2 and 1845-6.

He was anxious to introduce full-scale mechanisation as quickly as possible, and for his technical adviser he found a man in Reading who was an engineer with an enquiring and speculative nature similar to his own. William Exall was senior partner in Barrett, Exall & Andrewes' foundry which later became the Reading Iron Works Ltd. By mid-1846 their joint experiments had progressed so far that George Palmer was able to transfer his operations to a disused factory which already had a 25 h.p. steam engine. This was adapted by the ironworks to power the various machines by overhead shafts and endless bands.

The dough mixing took him some years to mechanise satisfactorily, but by 1851 he had two separate types of machine in regular use. One type mixed the hard dough for plain biscuits in drums that were smaller copies of Sir Thomas Grant's invention. Thus although the latter mixed 5 cwt. of dough in two minutes, the Reading drums dealt with 280 lbs., the contents of a normal sack of flour, in fifteen minutes. The other mixer was for the more malleable dough, softened by fancy ingredients such as butter, eggs, milk and flavouring that ranged from caraway to cinnamon, essence of lemon and orange-flower water. It was an open pan, into which the mixing shafts descended vertically and which was operated by a man who periodically stirred the mixture in order to keep it circulating.

One of the two rolling and cutting machines dealt with the hard dough and was known as the Captain's biscuit machine, while the other was the Cracknel machine for the softer dough. Although perhaps not unlike the ones at Carlisle, they did have as a special feature a reversible gear: this allowed the dough to be reduced to the necessary thickness in one operation by rolling it successively backwards and forwards. An endless band carried the dough under the cutters. The uncooked biscuit shapes fell off the end of the band on to trays, which were then wheeled off in trolleys to the ovens.

For baking George Palmer at first used hand ovens, 16 to 40 feet in depth, heated from below so as to minimise dust. However, his ultimate plan was to introduce a travelling oven; that is, one with moving parts that allowed the biscuits to travel slowly during the whole of the baking process. As it happened, the first patent for this had been taken out as long before as 1788, and in 1810 an oven had actually been built by

Admiral Sir Isaac Coffin (1759-1839), a Bostonian who made his career with the Royal Navy. Coffin's 'perpetual oven', as he called it in his patent, was 50 feet long and ran on a moving endless band of wire 3 feet wide. Unfortunately the cast-iron rollers and part of the band lay outside the oven and the consequent heat loss made it impracticable.[7]

George Palmer's initial search threw up two other interesting ideas, both protected by patents. A directly heated revolving oven was owned by the Patent Desiccating Co. of London and a hot air oven by a Liverpool firm. Although the moving parts of both were enclosed to conserve heat, he rejected both of them, and not until 1851 did he discover exactly what he wanted. That was a revolving oven, developed for ship's biscuits by William & Maxwell Scott of Tranmere near Liverpool. Measuring 20 feet long by 4½ feet wide, it contained a feeding web on which boys placed the uncooked biscuits. The shafting moved the web in a series of jerks so that after five to fifteen minutes, depending on the variety being baked, the biscuit would emerge through a screen that was just wide enough to allow it through without undue loss of heat.

These developments in ovens came none too soon, for by 1850-51 the value of the firm's sales was just five times that of 1846-7. Thus the baking could now be speeded up in line with the greater rapidity of the earlier processes. Instead of each oven having to be filled and emptied by hand every quarter of an hour or so, a whole succession of biscuits could be put through in a continuous flow. George Palmer's efforts over a period of ten years had thus reached fruition. Although he and his descendants went on to promote further inventions for many decades, with the adoption of this oven the pioneering age of biscuit-making came to an end.

The Consequences of Mechanisation

Despite the gaps in our evidence, we can trace with some assurance the way in which mechanisation contributed to forming the biscuit industry as we know it today. Demand for ship's biscuits continued to increase until towards the end of the nineteenth century bread could be successfully baked at sea and Board of Trade regulations made the installation of bread ovens compulsory on most vessels. One of the most noteworthy recruits to the industry after these innovations was Peek Frean & Co., established at Bermondsey in London during 1857. Although primarily a fancy biscuit specialist, about half its output comprised ship's biscuits. An interesting example of the latter being used as emergency rations was in 1871 when the French government ordered from Peek Frean and other British firms over 16,000 tons to feed the survivors of the long drawn-out siege of Paris. The growth of the army biscuit, for rather similar purposes of sustinence, from the South African War of 1899-1902 onwards, falls outside the scope of the present paper.

Huntley & Palmer, which never made ship's biscuits and therefore was not involved in the order from France, over the years to 1900 derived greater financial benefit than any of its competitors from the technical advances in fancy biscuit making. In the 1870s, for instance, it was the largest biscuit manufactory in the world. Then in 1898, after George Palmer's death, it became a limited company with a capital of £2,400,000, about ten times the capital of Carr & Co., Ltd., established at Carlisle in 1894; Carr's £253,000 capital included about £100,000 for the flour milling business that was hived off into a separate company in 1908. Our only other basis of comparison between the Reading and the Carlisle firms is the evidence that George Palmer gave to the jury of the Amsterdam exhibition in 1869. Such testimony in the nature of things tends to be one-sided; yet he was a Quaker and a singularly honest man, and some credence should therefore be given to it.

He looked both at the characteristics of the biscuits themselves and at those of the machines. As to the biscuits, at the time he was writing, Carr's produced only two varieties, the oblong ones from the printing press and the round ones from the rotary cutters, whereas even before 1841 his own firm had produced 30 kinds. Nor, according to him, had Carr's biscuits 'held their ground'. He also asserted that all competing firms 'though not entirely are in degree indebted to us for the types of biscuit and very largely for the distinguishing names of their biscuits', such as the Ginger Nut and Osborne. Since by the 1860s Huntley & Palmer produced some 120 varieties, far more than any rival, it seems reasonable to accept his point. As to the machines themselves, he did not dispute the priority of the Carlisle ones, but emphasised that those had never come into general use. They thus differed from his own, which had in fact encouraged a development vital to the emergence of an industry: the growth of specialist machinery suppliers. To quote once again from his 1869 submission, in 1846 'there was no engineering establishment in England where machines for the manufacture of fancy biscuits could be purchased'. Barrett, Exall & Andrewes' iron works did make a biscuit machine a few years later, which it entered for the London exhibitions of 1851 and 1862. The machine linked together the dough-mixing, rolling and cutting processes by means of endless bands: perhaps the first time that this had been done completely. However, the iron works found itself too greatly involved in agricultural machinery and steam engines to take on this speciality. That was left to another Liverpool firm, T. & T. Vicars, founded in 1849. According to an authoritative account, Vicars' partners 'early in their career had their attention drawn to the system of machinery for bread and biscuit baking, and in 1852 they took out their first patent for a better form of bread-baking oven'.[8] By then a firm of heating engineers, A.M. Perkins & Son, had begun to produce its own type of oven. Both firms' ovens were suitable for biscuits also, and they were drawn from that to mechanising the earlier processes of biscuit manufacture also.

Dr. Andrew Ure, in his *Dictionary of Arts, Manufactures and Mines* of 1853, singled out the Perkins hot-water oven as one of the two best available biscuit ovens. On the other hand, the *Encyclopaedia Britannica* of 1875 described Vicars as 'the chief manufacturers of biscuit machinery' and stated that its trade list mentioned no fewer than 128 different varieties of cutters.[9] A decade later Vicars itself was claiming most of the 'eminent biscuit baking firms' in Britain had adopted its patents in one form or another, while it had fulfilled orders to an impressive number of overseas firms, including ones in the United States. Even more interesting competition sprang up after 1878 with the establishment of Joseph Baker & Son, which by 1900 had become the most considerable machinery manufacturers in the whole of Britain's food industry. Among its specialities in the biscuit line were machines for macaroons and sugar wafers. In 1920 the Baker and the Perkins firms amalgamated into what later became Baker Perkins Ltd. Together with Vicars they remain the country's specialists in biscuit machinery.

The Creation of a Biscuit Industry

We have now seen one example of the emerging pattern of an industry proper: the appearance of specialist machinery suppliers, and further examples will be quoted in the present section. The first one to be considered is the growing consultation of member firms with one another about such matters as prices and discounts granted to customers. Indeed, they began to correspond as early as the 1840s, and not unexpectedly looked up to Huntley & Palmer as the price leader and main confidant. In 1849 and 1850 Carr's of Carlisle anxiously wrote to George Palmer several times about prices and the like, and complained about the way in which a London firm, Hill & Jones, was undercutting both their firms' prices. George Palmer merely advised Carr's to write direct and persuade Hill & Jones to 'play fair and not cut up the trade'. He himself had already used a number of commission agents to recruit reputable family grocers up and down the country as outlets for his biscuits, so that by then he had well over 700 retailers in nearly 400 different towns throughout the British Isles. Moreover, although Carr's had merely a small office in London, his own brother Samuel Palmer set up Huntley & Palmer's London office which took charge of the trade throughout the metropolis and also overseas. Carr's, he already knew, was not at all selective about what outlets it used, and that inevitably harmed its goodwill and by contrast strengthened his own firm's standing.

One consequence for the industry that did not occur was any marked increase in the productivity of its labour, as had happened with ship's biscuits. Instead, manufacturers preferred to bring out more and more different brands, either invented by themselves or copied from others: clearly an indispensable step as long as biscuits remained expensive products subject to the vagaries of public taste. By 1900 Huntley & Palmer had 400 different varieties and Peek Frean over half that number; how many Carr's then produced is not known. In firms such as Huntley & Palmer, directors with a mechanical bent would try their hands at devising ever more exotic types of biscuit. A remarkable and very successful example was the Breakfast biscuit, invented by the collaboration of George Palmer's sons, one an engineer and the other a scientist, since there were unprecedented problems in introducing yeast into a biscuit. But Peek Frean could claim comparable successes with more straightforward types, such as the Garibaldi, the Marie and (in the early twentieth century) the ever popular Pat-a-Cake.

However, other firms preferred to turn out a much smaller and more standardised range of biscuits at markedly cheaper prices, using less expensive ingredients and machinery bought from one or other of the suppliers. The Co-operative Wholesale Society, for instance, began to make biscuits at Crumpsall near Manchester in 1873; it was able to economise even further by using women and boys on lighter jobs traditionally reserved for men at Reading. The multiple grocers which sprang up in that decade, such as Liptons and the Home & Colonial Stores, soon made arrangements, either through setting up factories or by outside contracts, for making their own brands of biscuits. Since each of these cheap manufacturers had its own retail outlets, they saved on expenses like advertising and the use of representatives. By the turn of the century they were beginning to prove a definite threat to the expansion of the high-quality manufacturers, at a time when the latter might have been able to take advantage of steadily rising incomes, which allowed middle-class people to enjoy semi-luxuries that had earlier been outside their range.

In the nineteenth century, the top firms reacted in a very positive way to the competition by their cheaper rivals and by the Scottish and Irish manufacturers such as McVitie & Price, Macfarlane Lang and Jacob's of Dublin, which during the 1880s began to impinge on the English market by large-scale production with the aid of newly-installed machinery. Huntley & Palmer and Peek Frean then began to collaborate formally by exchanging advance information on matters of common interest so as to avoid wasteful price or discount wars between themselves. That did not prevent them from competing in other ways, for instance by aggressive advertising and the active promotion of new brands. They both decided to remain outside the

Association of Biscuit Manufacturers. This trade association had been set up in 1903, partly as a counterweight to the powerful Grocers Federation, and partly because several Scottish manufacturers had set up branch factories in England and had thus caused over-capacity in the industry just when demand had been hit by a deepening recession. Not until the end of the First World War, after all firms had been thrown together by common wartime problems and official regulations, did these two firms join a reconstituted and enlarged National Association of Biscuit Manufacturers.

Changing Patterns of Demand

This important aspect has been left until last, because the dietary changes to be considered took place some years after the pioneering developments in technology mentioned above. Contemporary literature indicates a rather limited role for the fancy biscuit in the very early days of the industry. A possible reason is that before the 1840s to 1860s well-to-do people enjoyed heavy breakfasts, often as late as 10 a.m., and had dinner at the early time of 4 to 5 p.m. This left little room for luncheon which even if taken was an informal cold meal and might be replaced by some wine at midday. Tea and cakes could be served in the late evening, or alternatively a light supper. Thus the Londoner Mr. Jorrocks consumed a few ship's biscuits — perhaps plain biscuits given that generic name — during his large hunting breakfasts, and the ladies of Knutsford, in Cheshire (thinly disguised as Cranford) nibbled a ladies' biscuit with their mid-morning wine, while those in Reading had Quaker-made biscuits during luncheon there: yet all these examples do not suggest much of a demand for biscuits, at least for daytime use. There was greater scope in the evenings. At Knutsford, Savoy and sponge biscuits were served at evening parties, and in the greatest of all Jane Austen's novels Mr. Woodhouse and Mrs. Bates sat down in his dining-room to tea and biscuits, sweetbread and asparagus, baked apples and wine — although as our informant is the garrulous Miss Bates, she does not make clear whether this comprised one meal or two.[10]

Such biscuits as were eaten, then, might have been made at home or bought from local pastrycooks; yet factory-made biscuits when they came in still proved expensive. Huntley & Palmers' Rout biscuit, for formal parties, cost 2s. (10p) a pound and Ratafias, Lemon and Orange Dessert and Raspberry biscuits more than 1s. (5p) a pound. Even ordinary varieties of the Ginger Nut and Osborne kind sold at 6d. (2½p), a quarter of what many labourers earned in a day. Nevertheless, as time went on there were enough customers with adequate incomes to buy from their family grocers or direct from the manufacturers in 1859 no less than 6 million lbs. of Huntley &

Palmer's and another million lbs. of Peek Frean's biscuits. These customers included members of the aristocracy and the gentry, as well as prelates and the more affluent clergy and institutions such as Oxford and Cambridge colleges, public schools and gentlemen's clubs. Typical as they were of the higher income groups, these categories still represented no more than a narrow section of the total population.

Then by the 1860s they had radically altered their mealtimes.[11] Breakfasts were served earlier, usually between 8 and 9, on a far less elaborate scale, and dinner time was put back until, say 7 – 8 p.m. That provided room for a set luncheon, and afternoon tea also became quite common: at both these meals biscuits were often served, plain ones of the Captain's variety with cheese at luncheon and sweet ones at teatime. Such changes probably spread from London to areas of affluence elsewhere in England, as their inhabitants chose to live further out from city centres and the menfolk became involved in commerce and industry. The number of men who were leisured or able to fit their occupations to the old-fashioned mealtimes steadily diminished; the decline in agriculture and landowning generally as the sole livelihood of a gentleman made it commoner for him to find something to do outside the home involving regular attendance at a place of work. Other contributing factors may have been the spread of day schools, first for boys and later on for girls, and the increasing mobility of women for visiting and shopping purposes. By the late 1870s Huntley & Palmer had doubled their productive capacity with a whole new complex of factory buildings and its output was as high as 37 million lbs., with Peek Frean contributing a further 17 million lbs.

The trend towards more biscuit eating was encouraged by certain changes below stairs. The quality, if not the number, of domestic servants had in their employers' opinions been declining almost ever since time began: as early as 1470 Jane Stonor in Oxfordshire was complaining that 'servants be not as diligent as they were wont to be'.[12] However, by the 1860s some efforts were being made to reduce the time wasted in the most skilled domestic occupation, namely cooking. Fewer products were home-made once similar articles could be bought at less cost outside, and ready-made foodstuffs in packets, such as custard and egg powders and shredded suet, began to reach the kitchen. The gradual dawn of the convenience food was breaking, and the biscuit as the most convenient of them all was likely to benefit as much as any.

Clearly the trends described above affected only well-to-do households: the less affluent have always eaten at hours to fit in with their employers' exacting demands. However, poor people were also finding certain perceptible changes occurring in their eating patterns. From the 1840s onwards, for instance, consumption per head of tea and sugar in Britain steadily rose, and in 1900 was over five times as high as in 1840. That was due to a progressive fall in their prices. Real wage rates, too, showed a distinct increase even allowing for unemployment.

Such developments gave to ordinary people at least the opportunity of wider choices of foodstuffs than in the past. Indeed, according to an authoritative source, 'there is a good case for selecting the 1880s as one of the decisive periods in the improvement of the standard of living of the working classes'.[13] It would be wrong to carry this point too far, as even at the end of the century average working-class budgets showed pitifully small sums expended on biscuits and cakes. Even so, the 6 million lbs. sold by the Co-operative Stores in Britain and the substantial trade by the multiple grocers in their own brands show that biscuits were already penetrating at least some way down the social scale.

Perhaps it would be permissible to stray yet again outside the limits of the nineteenth century to mention another noteworthy change in nutrition that occurred during and after the First World War. By then the increasing pace of normal life, together with a reaction against the heavy Victorian and Edwardian meals and the cults of slimming, vitamins and outdoor activities, stimulated an enormous and long unsatisfied demand for snacks and light convenience foods of all kinds. Those included fresh fruit, milk, nuts and of course biscuits. Evidence that the demand for biscuits is nowadays at last being met is that in 1939 the industry produced about 300,000 tons in all, but in 1974 produced over double that quantity, namely 628,000 tons.

Conclusion

The significance of the fancy biscuit in the social and industrial developments of the past 150 years or so in Britain has so far been somewhat underestimated by scholars researching in this field. Many gaps still remain in the evidence to hand. Even so, in this paper it has seemed worth while to set down what we know, in the hopes of stimulating further research some time in the future.

Notes

1. The present article is a revised and extended version of the paper read to the seminar on 10 December 1971, which was later incorporated into Chapter 4, 'Origins of Biscuit Manufacture', of the author's *Quaker Enterprise in Biscuits: Huntley & Palmers of Reading, 1822-1972,* 1972.
2. Figure of 'net output' from *Report of the Census of Production,* HMSO, 1972.
3. *Transactions of the Society of Arts,* XL, (1833-5), pp.97ff., and Peter Barlow, *Encyclopaedia of Manufacturers,* 1836, pp.801ff., also *Penny Magazine,* 4 April 1840, pp. 130-32.
4. On this point see the strong words about the 'adulteration of taste' and 'how ancient instincts were warped' through the mechanisation of bread-baking in S. Giedion, *Mechanization Takes Command,* New York, 1948, pp.200-1.
5. No satisfactory account has yet been published of J.D. Carr's invention. A useful description of his factory is given in *Chambers' Edinburgh Journal,* No. 135, New Series, 1 August 1846.
6. References to events in Huntley & Palmer can be found in the author's book mentioned in fn. 1 above.
7. Giedion, *Mechanization Takes Command,* pp.176ff. and 190ff.
8. *Royal Album of Arts, Manufactures and Mines,* I, pp.343ff. s.v. 'Biscuits', references to the Baker and Perkins firms see Augustus Muir, *The History of Baker Perkins,* 1968, esp. pp.10ff.
9. A. Ure, *Dictionary of Arts Manufactures and Mines,* I, pp.343ff. s.v. 'Biscuits', and *Encyclopaedia Britannica,* 1875, III, pp.252ff., s.v. 'Baking'.
10. R.S. Surtees, *Jorrocks' Jaunts and Jollities,* Everyman's Edition, 1928, p.58; Mrs. Gaskell, *Cranford,* World's Classics, 1916, pp. 4, 10, 31, 80 and 166; M.R. Mitford, *Belford Regis,* reprinted 1942, pp.108 and 275; and Jane Austen, *Emma,* R.W. Chapman (ed.), 1923, p.329. The last-named corrects the statement in *Quaker Enterprise in Biscuits,* p.51, that there is only one reference to biscuits in Jane Austen's novels.
11. J. Burnett, *Plenty and Want,* 1966, pp.54-5, seems to place the transition a decade earlier, from the 1830s onwards, but the evidence is conflicting. See G.M. Young (ed.), *Early Victorian England 1830-65,* 1934, pp. 90ff., and Arnold Palmer, *Movable Feasts,* 1952, pp.70ff.
12. C.L. Kingsford (ed.), *The Stonor Letters and Papers 1290-1483,* I, Camden 3rd Series XXIX, 1919, p.110.
13. J. Burnett, *Plenty and Want,* p.92.

3 THE 'CONSUMER REVOLUTION' AND THE GROWTH OF FACTORY FOODS: CHANGING PATTERNS OF BREAD AND CEREAL-EATING IN BRITAIN IN THE TWENTIETH CENTURY

E.J.T. COLLINS

Since 1900, the demand for cereal foods, which historically were a mainstay of human dietary, has been affected by changes in real incomes and by the forces of the 'consumer revolution' (see Table I).

Table I: *The food share of consumer expenditure 1900-65*[1]
(percentage at current prices)

1900-09	1910-19	1920-29	1930-39	1940-49	1950-59	1960-65
28.5	30.9	31.4	27.4	23.5	26.7	23.7

Cereals moving into consumption in the UK 1900-70
(in lbs. per head per annum)

1909-13	1924-28	1934-38	1941	1944	1950	1960	1970
237	214	210	257	253	223	181	160

Cereal expenditure as a percentage of total food expenditure

1900-09	1910-19	1920-29	1930-39	1940-49	1950-59	1960-69
16.0	17.0	14.6	14.6	17.9	16.4	15.3

The pattern in 1900 — wheaten flour and white bread, with cakes and biscuits semi-luxuries, the output of manufactured cereal foods small and unimportant and oatmeal porridge popular only in the higher income groups and in Scotland — was tedious and unexciting compared with a century earlier when cereals were eaten in many different forms — wet, dry, hot, cold, baked, griddled — and when there was much local and regional variety in the colour and composition of the household loaf.[2] Since 1900 the trend has been one of increasing diversification, characterised by a switch from the cheaper more traditional foods to the costlier and more highly formulated foods. The overall result has been a fall in the proportions of both the weight and the value of bread and flour to total cereal consumption.

Bread

The price and income elasticity of demand for bread has been lower than for most other major categories of foodstuffs, and since 1900 it has become an 'inferior good', in the sense that consumption has fallen as real incomes have risen. The reasons are well known and require no repetition beyond emphasising the importance of changes in eating habits (e.g. the decline of the 'packed lunch' and 'afternoon tea'), of the demand for lighter and more savoury foods, and the many social factors, grounded in the 'consumer revolution', which streamlined the domestic routine.[3] Bread consumption between the wars may have levelled off because of the increasing popularity of the sandwich, and although bread-eating reached new peaks during and immediately after the Second World War, consumption had already fallen below pre-war levels by 1953, and thereafter sank rapidly. The National Food Survey suggests a 30 per cent fall between 1950 and 1970, from 55 oz. to 36 oz. per week, and a rate of decline spread more or less evenly across the different income groups. But although *per capita* consumption has fallen, the industrial production of bread is still very much higher today than in 1920, as a result partly of population growth and partly of the decline of home-baking (in 1920 loose flour represented about 25 per cent of wheaten flour sales compared with 14 per cent in the late sixties.[4] The greater expansion, however, was in flour confectionery, whose production rose from 35 per cent of bakery sales in 1924 to 46 per cent in 1954.[5]

These trends must be seen against the broader background of structural change in the bakery industries. A major development which began about 1930 was the displacement of the small master baker by the large plant bakery. In 1937 plant bakeries were responsible for only 10–12 per cent of national bread output, but by 1953 the proportion had increased to 35–40 per cent, and by the late sixties to about 70 per cent.[6] The economics of plant bakeries were those of mass production, economies of scale and vertical integration into the retail trades.[7] Multiple-shop bakeries began in the nineteenth century with the co-operative movement and by 1939 over 30 per cent of bread sales were channelled through about 2,400 shops owned by just 79 firms.[8] Allied Bakeries, founded in 1935 by Garfield Weston, was the first private firm to distribute bread nationally, and by 1938 it owned directly or through its subsidiaries 28 bakeries and 217 shops. Between 1953 and 1956 it acquired a further 10 bakeries including the Aereated Bread Company and its 165 ABC tea-shops, and at the end of the decade controlled about 18 per cent of the national bread trade.[9] This trend has accelerated since the early 1950s as falling bread consumption has intensified the plant bakery's need to ensure that its trade is large enough to keep its plants busy and as the milling interest has sought downstream markets for its meals and flours. Today, just four firms, Associated British Foods, Spillers, Ranks Hovis McDougall and the CWS control about 70 per cent of national bread production.[10] Meanwhile, the numbers of master bakers have fallen from more than 20,000 in 1900 to less than 10,000 today. Of the survivors, some have ceased bread-making altogether, while others have concentrated on the manufacture of 'crusty' and 'fancy' breads, and on flour confectionery, especially 'morning goods' and other more perishable wares whose short shelf-life and high distribution costs render them less suitable for plant-bakery production.[11] The advantages of the large bakeries have been most apparent in the production of slab cake and sliced and ready-wrapped bread, which found a ready market in the grocery chain stores. Since 1950 the decline, through rising costs, of door-to-door delivery, and the growth of the supermarket, have broken the monopoly of the specialised distributor.[12] The 1961 Census of Distribution recorded 148,230 shops selling bread and flour confectionery of which approximately three-quarters were grocery and provision dealers.[13]

The chief limiting factor in the growth of the bread market has been falling *per capita* consumption. Advertising has had little effect on demand other perhaps than to redistribute brand shares, either in the 1930s or, more recently, through the generic advertising campaigns organised by the Flour Advisory Bureau.[14] The alternative course — that of expansion through diversification — has proved almost as unrewarding. Failure to diversify can be attributed to the nature of the product, which is unique and has few direct substitutes, and implied in this, the technical constraints which limit product innovation to minor changes in shape, appearance, colour and composition. Except for wrapping and slicing (which came in between the wars) and the bread roll, it has little appeal as a convenience food, while the falling demand for jams and preserves (by 25 per cent *per capita* between 1958 and 1970) suggests that its potential as a snack food may also have been exhausted.[15]

These factors apart, perhaps the most severe constraint, even within the fairly narrow limits of product design and manufacture, has been the strength of consumer preference for a single product, the white wheaten loaf, which comprised in 1900 over 95 per cent and in 1970 still over 80 per cent of bread consumption by weight.[16] Speciality and patent breads first appeared in the 1880s and by 1912 a few, such as Hovis (reinforced wheat germ), Daren (wheat, ryemeal and wheat germ), Kermode's (wheat and maize), Triagon (wheat, maize and rice) and Malt Loaf, had acquired a regional or national reputation.[17] The range now includes 'high-protein' and 'low-calorie' breads and also crispbread (strictly a biscuit and a bread substitute) which was introduced between the wars as a slimming food (the firm of Ryvita opened its Birmingham factory in the 1930s).[18] The main competition, however, was between white breads and brown breads, which latter, made from low-extraction flours, were virtually extinct in Britain in 1850, but were reintroduced, primarily as health foods, in the last quarter of the nineteenth century. Yet after many years of exhortation and advice by food scientists and health reformists as to its superior nutritive value, the brown bread share of the national bread market is today still less than 10 per cent.[19]

The difficulties in breaking down a consumer preference of this order can be illustrated, by way of digression, from the history of the firm of Hovis Limited which, since the 1890s, has been the UK market leader in brown bread.[20] Hovis is a firm of millers manufacturing a patent flour which is sold to the bakery trade. The special feature of Hovis flour is its super-high concentration of wheat germ which in ordinary flours is removed in the milling process. The idea may have owed something to the American vegetarian Sylvester Graham, who invented a triturated bran loaf in the 1840s, but the present formula was patented about 1885 by Richard Smith, a miller at Stone, Staffordshire, who, in 1887, sold the rights to another milling firm, Fitton and Sons of Macclesfield. In 1891, after a national competition, the flour was renamed Hovis, from the Latin construction, 'hominus vis', strength of man, and in 1898, out of the new trade mark, the Hovis Bread Company was founded.

The product was locally successful and, in 1896, it was decided to increase production and expand the market into the larger centres of population. In that year the company purchased the Imperial Mills at Westminster, and later, in 1906, erected a new mill at Trafford Park, Manchester. Subsequently, additional mills, flour and provender were acquired in other parts of the country, at ports and in wheat-producing areas, until by 1939 Hovis controlled between 7 and 8 per cent of national flour output.[21] The problems though, were not of supply, but of demand — of winning the confidence of the public and the support of the bakery trade. Thus, it was necessary to campaign simultaneously at each main link in the chain of manufacture and distribution. The baker was won over by the offer of a nationally advertised branded product together with a wide range of supporting services. In 1895 a printing plant was set up at Macclesfield to produce leaflets, billheads, advertisement cards, paper bags, cardboard boxes, bread bins and delivery baskets, all of which carried a Hovis advertisement, for sale to the trade at competitive prices. In 1905 these activities were extended to include the design and manufacture of signs and sign boards for bakers' vans and barrows. The van departments, the first of which was established in London in Buckingham Palace Road, began later to undertake van repair work and actual van-building, which not only increased the company's share of in-trade advertising but was also a valuable source of income between the wars when door-to-door delivery by motor lorry and electric van became the vogue. The Company also provided the baker with special baking tins, each with the Hovis imprint, which he was obliged to use when making Hovis bread, and which was a successful first attempt, prior to the introduction of the wrapped loaf, at brand-naming. As well, it organised, from the 1890s, a programme of regional and national baking competitions to improve standards of Hovis bread-making and to popularise the art and the product.

In the approach to the consumer, the aim throughout has been to overcome the popular prejudice against the brown loaf by emphasising product benefits. In the early years the goal was to acquire a sound reputation with a public that was sceptical of patent foods and wary of adulteration. Thus early advertisements made considerable play of royal patronage, of awards and diplomas for quality and purity, and of the need to beware cheap imitations. Hovis was depicted as a health food — as a cure for indigestion and source of 'good bone, brain, flesh and muscle' — conveyed by the messages 'Hovis builds strong men', 'Keep the wolf from the door' and 'England's pride and England's glory'. Initially, press advertising was centred on quality journals and magazines like *Strand, Black & White* and *Illustrated London News,* but in 1906, in a bid to broaden the base of the market, several advertisements, ranging to full front-page spreads, were placed in national daily newspapers, such as the *Graphic* and *Daily Mail.*

By 1914 the trade mark had become a household word, and a base had been built from which to launch the intensive promotional campaigns of the inter-war years. Hovis employed simultaneously several different techniques, directed at different sections of the market and at different susceptibilities. Brash 'cartoon-ads' — in 1926 even a cartoon film — competed with pseudo-scientific advertisements aimed at creating in the mind of the consumer a dietary problem which only Hovis could resolve. 'Do you', asked one advertisement, 'buy a loaf by its colour or by its food value?' Hovis identified itself more positively with the *sans corpa* through its association with the 'Fitter Britain Movement' and with Thomas Inch, the muscle-man, and author of many books and pamphlets on health, diet and body-building. In-store and in-trade advertising were carried on under the cloak of services to the bakery trade. Outdoor advertising was liberally spread over vans, buses, railway stations, roadside hoardings and at cafes and restaurants. The growing public interest in hiking, motoring and cycling brought in its wake a rash of country tea-shops, and with them, 'Teas with Hovis' signs, and special tea-sets, which were a Hovis novelty in 1900, but found a perfect niche in the mock-Tudor world of the 1930s. Since the Second World War, advertising appropriations have been spent more narrowly, and today, as part of the Ranks Hovis McDougall group, most of the budget is allocated to television, which has displaced the press as the main advertising channel for proprietary foods.

The firm of Hovis has been a major force in the modern food industry, but at no point has its share of the total bread market exceeded 5 per cent. It is, though, a measure of achievement that since 1950 the level of brown bread consumption per head has been maintained where that of white bread has fallen. Up to the Second World War brown bread was a predominantly upper-income food; a 1936 survey records that average consumption in income groups A and B was more than three times greater than in income groups C and D.[22] Since 1950 the gap has closed, to the point — which raises interesting speculations as to future trends in demand — that consumption is now highest in income group D households, and highest of all among Old Age Pensioners.[23]

The Origins of Breakfast Cereals

Ready-to-eat (RTE) breakfast cereals had the style and versatility that the bread foods had not. They originated in the United States in the second half of the nineteenth century.[24] They were developed to meet the needs of vegetarian groups like the Seventh Day Adventists who, at Battle Creek, Michigan, were already experimenting with cereal-based foods in the 1850s, and later, of dietary reformists who were an important market for patent foods. The concept and formulation of breakfast cereals owed much to the work of Dr. John Harvey Kellogg, the Director of the 'medical boarding house' (later the Sanitarium) at Battle Creek, where he researched into the 'dietary problem' and the development of so-called 'natural foods'. In the 1860s he formulated 'Granola', the first ready-cooked breakfast cereal food, made from a mixture of wheat, oatmeal and maize baked in a slow oven until thoroughly dextrinised. In 1896 he produced 'Granose', the first flaked cereal food, made of wheat, and three years later, by the same process, the inimitable corn flake. Kellogg also helped to popularise the science of applied dietetics and to stimulate experimental work elsewhere on patent cereal foods. By the 1890s many minds were bent to the same problem, and the decade around 1895 saw in quick succession the development of most of the basic types of pre-cooked cereal and manufacturing process (i.e. flaking, toasting, puffing and extrusion). Shredded Wheat was invented in 1892 by Henry D. Perky of Denver; Grape Nuts in 1898 by Charles W. Post (an ex-patient of Kellogg's at the Sanitarium); Puffed Wheat in 1902 by Alexander Anderson, and Toasted Oat Flakes, again in the 1890s, by the Beck Cereal Company of Detroit. These discoveries plunged the American Midwest into something of a breakfast cereal boom, but of the many inventions, few survived the outbreak of the Great War. By 1920 the less efficient producers had been forced out of business, and control of the market has passed into the hands of a few large firms headed by Kellogg, the Force Food Company of Buffalo, the Shredded Wheat Company of

Niagara Falls (now part of National Biscuit), Quaker Oats, Armour Grain of Chicago (now the Ralston Purina Company) and the Postum Cereals Company (now the Post Division of General Foods).

The factors underlying the successful intrusion of breakfast cereals into the North American and British dietary patterns were complex. Though conceived originally as health foods, their success in the longer run was due to other, more dynamic forces, such as rising real incomes, changing patterns of work and employment and the overall quickening tempo of twentieth-century living, which created a niche for lighter and quicker foods. There were other important influences. Special opportunities for product design and innovation were afforded by the uniquely twentieth-century phenomenon of the children's market, at which, after 1920, the main promotional effort was directed. The numbers of working wives were growing, and convenience foods, especially in the early morning, became a part of the domestic routine.

Many of the early pioneers of the breakfast cereals industry had been motivated by an interest in dietetics, but it was vigorous salesmanship that convinced the public at large that breakfast cereals were a utility food and not just a 'health food oddity'. Charles Post, the inventor of Grape Nuts and Post Toasties, was the first to apply the symptom-inducing advertising techniques used by the makers of patent medicines. In pioneering the art of 'selling health foods to well people', he widened the appeal of scientific eating and anticipated the important role that the food industry was to play in stimulating (and focusing) public interest in health and nutrition. W.K., brother of John Harvey, established the Kellogg Co. as world leader through skilful advertising and single-minded concentration on the large popular markets in the American cities.[25] The year 1906 saw the 'Wink at your Grocer' campaign; 1907, the first 'Sweetheart of the corn' advertisement; 1912 the erection in Times Square of the world's largest illuminated sign, and the 1930s, in the face of depression and falling prices, the doubling of advertising expenditures, and expansion overseas. Brand image was embodied in catch-phrases like the 'Sunshine breakfast', 'Just a little bit better', 'The road to Wellville', and, most enduringly, 'The original has this signature'. The US breakfast cereals industry pioneered the wax-tite container and dynamic packaging. It evolved new techniques of product development, test and consumer-marketing and in-store promotion. Since the 1920s the trend in the industry has been towards higher levels both of product concentration (in 1950 five companies accounted for over 95 per cent of RTE sales), and of conglomeration (incorporating other food manufacturing interests such as pet foods, groceries and poultry).[26] In short, the achievement was the wholly formulated, socially engineered product, and an industry which in technology, research and development, promotional techniques and corporate structure, has exemplified modern food manufacturing.

The British Market for Breakfast Cereals

Cereal-based health and baby foods have been manufactured in Britain the late nineteenth century. In 1912 over sixty different brands of proprietary cereal foods are recorded, but few commanded a large following.[27] These included Falona (a mixture of wheat, oats, barley and bean flour) and John Bull (malted cereal and dried milk) as well as a number of North American products, imported either directly from the United States, or from Canada, through subsidiary companies of US firms. In 1893 the American Cereal Company, the forerunner of Quaker Oats, established an agency in London, and in 1899, a subsidiary company for the sale of rolled oats and later of Puffed Wheat, Muffets (a shredded wheat product) and Corn Flakes.[28] In 1902 A.C. Fincken of Watford was appointed UK distributor for Force Wheat Flakes, manufactured by the Force Food Company of Canada.[29] Shredded Wheat, made by the Shredded Wheat Company of Canada, was first imported by a firm of grocers in 1908, and shortly afterwards a UK subsidiary company was formed.[30] Apart from 'Granose', there is no direct evidence that Kellogg products were imported before the Great War, but both Grape Nuts (made by the Postum Cereals Company) and Malta Vita (made by the Battle Creek Pure Food Co.) were recorded in 1912.[31]

The assault proper on the UK market, and the subsequent rapid broadening of the market base, began after 1920 when a number of leading American firms set up manufacturing plants in this country. In 1920, Quaker opened a small factory at Ware in Hertfordshire to produce Puffed Wheat and Puffed Rice, and in 1936, a large modern factory at Southall, Middlesex, which produced a wider range of products, to include, eventually, Quaker Oats.[32] The Shredded Wheat Company started manufacturing at Welwyn Garden City in 1925.[33] Kellogg began to import Corn Flakes and All Bran in 1922 and Rice Krispies in 1929, and in 1938 opened its first UK factory at Trafford Park, Manchester.[34] The only major British enterprise, and that only partly so, because two of its three founders were South African while the product itself had Battle Creek and Seventh Day Adventist connections, was the African Cereal Company (now Weetabix Ltd.), which set up a factory in a run-down flour mill at Burton Latimer, in Northamptonshire, in 1932.[35] Indigenous enterprise was largely confined to the manufacture of porridge oats, which was carried on in numerous small mills up and down the country. Yet even here, as with other breakfast cereal foods, the industry was dominated by American firms. In the late 1930s Quaker controlled an estimated 62 per cent of the rolled oats market and Kellogg and Shredded Wheat over 80 per cent of the ready-cooked market.[36] Partly as a result of the war, during which imports of maize and rolled oats were reduced and imports of Force Wheat Flakes ceased altogether, production is now rather less concentrated, but porridge is still dominated by the two firms, Scotts and Quaker, and ready-cooked cereals by the four firms, Kellogg, Weetabix, Nabisco and Quaker, which in 1970 accounted for almost 90 per cent of sales by weight.[37]

The overall trends in the output and consumption of breakfast cereals are reasonably clear, but before 1950 difficult to quantify. Up to the Great War it may be assumed that the market for rolled oats expanded faster than that for RTE cereals, which were still a relatively high-cost speciality food. The RTE market grew dramatically between the wars, especially between 1936 and 1940 when Kellogg sales alone rose by nearly 80 per cent, and by the outbreak of war its value exceeded that of porridge oats.[38] In the Second World War the pattern of development was interrupted by a shortage of raw materials and by 'zoning schemes' which confined company sales to different parts of the country. Following the removal of wartime controls, the pre-war trend was resumed; consumption of RTE cereals rose continuously over the fifties and sixties while those of traditional porridge, from a peak in 1947, thereafter declined relatively and absolutely, in weight and value.

The total quantities of breakfast cereals entering the UK market can be calculated from production (retained home production + imports); from consumption (average consumption *per capita* × population), or directly, from retail sales. The evidence, however, is too patchy and unreliable for any one method to yield a continuous series for the whole of the period since 1900. The Board of Trade Censuses of Production did not separately distinguish 'breakfast cereals' until 1937-8 prior to which they were enumerated under the head of 'infant and invalid foods', or later, under that of 'farinaceous preparations', whose factory value was put at £2,276,000 in 1935.[39] A further difficulty is that up to the 1930s a high proportion of breakfast cereal foods — porridge and RTE — was imported from North America, and was not separately recorded in the Annual Trade and Navigation Accounts. 'Breakfast cereal food in packets for retail sale' feature specifically in the post-war Censuses of Production but the results, (summarised in Appendix I), are not directly comparable and thus do not form a reliable series. Nor do they always tally with the (probably) more authentic figures, compiled by the firm of A.C. Nielson, of RTE sales through retail grocers, (Table II) although in some years (e.g. 1948 and 1968) their gross magnitudes roughly conform. The overall trend, post-war, is confirmed by the estimates of grain disposals in the UK from 1946-67 (see Appendix II).

With consumption we are on firmer ground in as much as there exist for the later 1930s a number of useful consumer surveys, and from 1940 onwards a more or less continuous series, compiled from official sources, of domestic food consumption and expenditure. Average consumption

Table II: *Total retail sales by weight of RTE breakfast cereals 1950-70*[40]
(in tons)

1950	1955	1961	1970	1971
64,500*	73,400*	95,800	132,900	134,500

*The original A.C. Nielson figures for these years excluded sales through co-operatives and were adjusted upwards for the purposes of the Monopolies Commission enquiry.

of RTE breakfast cereals in the UK in 1938 was estimated at 29 oz. per head of the population.[41] Consumption in working-class households rose, despite the war, to 38–42 oz. in 1942-45, and 62 oz. in 1950.[42] Between the early fifties and early seventies consumption doubled to nearly 150 oz. per head.[43] Conversely, the consumption of porridge oats which increased (or recovered) during the war due to food shortages and reached a peak in 1947-8 following the failure of the potato harvest, fell from 70 oz. in 1950 to 30 oz. in 1972, and in terms of value, from one-third to one-eighth of total expenditure on breakfast cereals.[44] (see Table III).

Table III: *Breakfast cereals: average consumption and expenditure 1938-72*[45]
(in ounces/pence per head per annum)

Consumption	1938	1942-45	1950	1960	1972
All breakfast cereals	74	90	142	143	179
RTE breakfast cereals	29	40	73	94	149
Oatmeal and oat products	45	50	69	49	30
Expenditure					
All breakfast cereals	–	56	103	199	389
RTE breakfast cereals	–	35	68	154	347
Oatmeal and oat products	–	21	35	45	42

The appeal of breakfast cereals lay in their palatability and convenience. The pattern of diffusion was, however, complex. Between the wars, ready-cooked breakfast cereals, oatmeal porridge and bacon and eggs competed directly with each other for pride of place on many middle and working-class breakfast tables. Consumer surveys, conducted in the 1930s, suggest a high price and income elasticity of demand for RTE cereals and bacon and eggs, and for both a significantly higher consumption in upper- than lower-income households.[46] In York, for example, a typical breakfast in the lowest income group was bread and dripping with a little bacon at weekends.[47] In southern Britain, where there was no long tradition of oatmeal-eating, porridge became popular in upper-class homes after 1870 and subsequently spread down the social scale. In Scotland, on the other hand, porridge was a traditional dish but its popularity was declining. Curious it was, that porridge had to cross the Atlantic and suffer a sea change before it became a utility food in England.[48] Before 1940 the pattern of change was, therefore, complicated. In the post-war period RTE cereals spread down and across the income scale, mainly at the expense of the hot breakfast. In 1936, according to the Crawford and Broadley survey, average expenditure on RTE cereals in income groups A and B was double that in Groups C and D, whereas in 1970 the income correlation, although still positive, was of a much smaller order.[49] The breakfast surveys of 1936, 1958, 1965 and 1967 show a progressive increase in the numbers of RTE eaters and suggest that by the late sixties ready-cooked cereals were the most popular weekday breakfast and that bacon and eggs were more usually reserved for weekends.[50] The decline of porridge-eating was a surrender to the convenience and for children especially, the frivolity of ready-cooked cereals. Rolled oats offered few opportunities for product innovation, so that technically, the different oatmeals competed with each other on speed of preparation. In 1922, at the same time as Armour Grain was announcing big price reductions on its corn flakes, Vernons were introducing their new three-minute 'Millenium' oats.[51] A new generation of 'instant porridges' was launched in 1965 but failed to arrest the slide and succeeded only in redistributing brand shares.[52]

Advertising

Breakfast cereals have always been associated with intensive advertising and vigorous promotion which, in their method and general strategy, followed much the same lines as in North America. Historically, advertising expenditures have been high, normally between 10 and 20 per cent of net sales, but in the case of the Kellogg Company as high as 28 per cent in the mid-1930s.[53] It is estimated that in 1935 some £700,000, or about 18 per cent of manufacturers' net sales, was spent on proprietary breakfast cereals, as compared with 2.6 per cent on self-raising flour; 2.3 per cent on biscuits and 2.0 per cent on bread.[54] In 1938 cereal foods were said to account for about 10 per cent of total food advertising expenditure, more than four-fifths of which was taken by the four firms, Kellogg, Quaker, Shredded Wheat and Postum Cereals.[55] The emphasis of promotional effort shifted over time as the size and composition of the market changed and as new media became available. The strategy employed today is different from that in 1930 when appropriations were spent mainly on dealer aids and on advertisements in the national press, and different again than at the turn of the century, when, at the two extremes, the emphases were on tasteful advertisement in the better-class magazines, and outrageous stunts like the draping of advertising banners across the face of the white cliffs of Dover.[56] Since the 1920s advertising has been aimed mainly at children and at the more aggressive sections of the grocery trade, notably chain stores and supermarkets.[57] The 1950s saw important developments, pioneered by Kellogg's, in 'dynamic packaging', and a rash of in-packet promotions such as competitions, back-panel cut-outs, mail-in-offers, self-liquidators and give-aways. In the sixties there was more stress on product benefits, and recently on more sophisticated types of advertisement aimed at adult audiences.

Yet despite the thrust and aggressiveness of the industry, and the novelty of its products, a main feature of the post-war RTE breakfast cereals market has been the relative conservatism of the consumer, so much so that today over 70 per cent of sales by weight comprise the old pre-war favourites, Corn Flakes, Shredded Wheat, Weetabix, and Puffed Wheat (Table IV).

Table IV: *Market shares of the main types of RTE breakfast cereals*[58]

	Percentage of homes using		Market shares by weight
	1939	1956	1970
Corn Flakes	64	56	39
Shredded Wheat	23	14	12
Weetabix	2	14	22
Puffed Wheat	4	14	2
Puffed Rice	2	NA	NA
Force Wheat Flakes	10	–	–
Other products	3	21	25

Since 1950 many attempts have been made to widen the appeal of breakfast cereals and steal marches over competitors by the introduction of new products, but with only limited success. In 1970 more than fifteen different products competed for a 25 per cent market share. Indeed, the road from Battle Creek is strewn with failures. One UK manufacturer test-marketed thirteen new products between 1953 and 1956, only three of which have endured, while an American firm, General Mills, failed spectacularly in its attempts to introduce into this country a range of products many of which were market leaders across the Atlantic.[59] In fact, successful introductions have tended to be not radically new products but variations on existing products, such as sugar-coated corn flakes and miniature shredded wheats. A constraint on product innovation has been the limitations of manufacturing techniques, the potential of which had already been largely exhausted by the early 1950s. Conversely, the most successful recent innovation, 'muesli', which was launched in 1972, has a simple formulation and can be cheaply and easily manufactured. The muesli example underlines the basic formula for success, that of distinctiveness of product plus efficient marketing. The costs of launching a new product are high. A recent study of breakfast cereals in the USA has shown that 56 months normally elapse between first activity and the stage of limited distribution and that most products, if they survived that long, broke even only in the third year of introduction.[60] These barriers have had the result, in the longer run, of narrowing the range of effective competition to relatively few products, with limited competition between the producers in the supply of like varieties. Today the Corn Flakes market is virtually monopolised by a single manufacturer whereas in the 1920s the consumer had a choice of at least six different brands.

Conclusion

The difference between bread and breakfast cereals was only in part material and technological. Above all, it was a difference in concept, between the traditional and socially engineered product, that was apparent at each and every link in the chain from manufacturer to consumer. Bread was an 'inferior good' and the brown bread experience suggests that the potential of new products is weak where the benefits are intangible and the incentives are not deeply grounded, socially or dietetically, in the 'consumer revolution'. These differences are further reflected in the structure of the two industries. In the one, concentration has been primarily associated with marketing efficiency and the development of brand names; in the other with manufacturing efficiency and control of the retail trade. In breakfast cereals there has been continuous product development and innovation, whereas bread had relatively little scope or opportunity for diversification.[61] The basis of competition in breakfast cereals was not just one of price because in the mind of the consumer each offering was 'a different bargain' distinguished by way of trade mark, design formulation, taste, colour, and utility. In the late 1930s an estimated £700,000 was spent on advertising breakfast cereals compared with only £170,000 on bread.[62] In the late 1960s maize and other edible raw materials represented 24 per cent, packing and packaging 20 per cent and advertising and promotion 12 per cent of the net sales value of Kellogg's Corn Flakes. In bread manufacture the respective values were of the approximate order:

40 per cent, 3–5 per cent and 1–2 per cent.[63]

Dietary change, like the standard of living itself, is a slippery concept. In 1929, J. Edgar Hoover analysed the essence of American prosperity as the stimulation and satisfaction of human wants to the point where 'the great mass of consumers will never for a moment know what it means to be content'.[64] This paper has suggested that role of the consumer in the growth of the modern food industry was rather more positive, and that changes in cereal-eating habits were the result of a more complex, and often unpredictable inter-reaction between supply and demand and between the market and the manufacturer.

Appendix I: *Census of production estimates of output of RTE breakfast cereals 1935-68*

A = thousand tons   B = thousand £

	Wheat Products		Maize Products		Other Products		Total Products	
	A	B	A	B	A	B	A	B
1935[1]	10	707	72[4]	3,897	–	–	82	4,604
1937[1]	12	825	73[4]	5,612	–	–	85	6,437
1948[2]	55	5,112	93	4,187	–	–	148	9,299
1951[2]	40[3]	4,811	117[5]	8,539	–	–	157	13,350
1954[2]	43	6,264	197[5]	12,419	–	–	240	18,683
1963[2]	53	11,230	58	12,665	52[6]	8,214	163	32,109
1968[2]	72	16,031	68	14,921	66	12,263	206	43,215

1. production only.
2. packeted for retail sale.
3. includes small quantities of milling offals.
4. the census records 718,000 and 733,000 tons in 1935-37 and I have assumed a one-place decimal error although the adjusted figures seem too high in view of the then still high volume of imported maize products.
5. includes 'other flaked maize'.
6. the basis of distinction between 'maize' and 'other' products is not clear, although the latter would have included some (few) barley and oats (excluding oatmeal) products which until 1963 were not enumerated separately.

Appendix II: *Grain disposals for use in the manufacture of breakfast cereal foods in the UK 1946-67*[1]

(in '000 tons)

	Wheat		Oats	Maize
1946/7 – 1950/1	8[2]	(1949)	294	47
1956/7 – 1960/1	–		154	98
1963/4	–		126	151
1966/7	75		118	c. 200

Sources: 1. D.K. Britton, *Cereals in the United Kingdom*, 1919, pp.513-15.
2. *Survey of agricultural, forestry and history products in the UK and their utilization*, Development Commission 1953, pp.6–8.

Notes

1. Derived from C.H. Feinstein, *National income, expenditure and output of the United Kingdom 1855-1965,* Cambridge, 1972, Table 25, whose data were derived from A.R. Prest and A.A. Adams, *Consumers' Expenditure in the United Kingdom, 1900-1919,* Cambridge, 1954, and R. Stone and D.A. Rowe, *The Measurement of Consumers' Expenditure and Behaviour in the United Kingdom, 1920-1938,* 2 vols., Cambridge, 1953 and 1966. 'Food' includes all household consumption of foods and non-alcoholic beverages, plus garden and allotment produce, valued at farm prices, but excludes consumption in hotels and restaurants, which, if included, would have raised the post-war (cf. pre-war) food fraction by about 2 per cent. In 1960 it was estimated that about £380 million was spent on 'meals and refreshments out' (J. Burnett, *Plenty & Want,* 1966, p.278). If we assume that turnover in the hotel and catering industry rose by an estimated 140 per cent over the next thirteen years (*Financial Times,* 8 June 1974) probably over £900 million was thus spent in 1973-74. J.C. McKenzie, 'Food trends, the dynamics of accomplished change', in J. Yudkin & J.C. McKenzie (eds.), *Changing Food Habits,* 1964, p.41; *Household Food Consumption and Expenditure,* 1970 and 1971, Ministry of Agriculture, Fisheries and Food, 1973, (serial together with Supplement of food expenditure by working-class households, 1940-49, which is bound with 1950 report, hereafter referred to as NFS – National Food Survey).
2. For nineteenth-century trends in cereal-eating, see, E.J.T. Collins, 'Dietary change and cereal consumption in Britain in the nineteenth century' (forthcoming, *Agricultural History Review*).
3. J. Yudkin & J.C. McKenzie (eds.), *Changing Food Habits,* 1964, pp.40-43; P. Maunder, *The Bread Industry in the United Kingdom,* Dept. Ag. Econ. Univ. Nottingham, and Dept. of Soc. Science and Econ., Univ. Technology, Loughborough, n.d., pp.15-21.
4. Stone & Rowe, op. cit., p.26; NFS, 1966-70.
5. Census of Production, 1935, op. cit., p.46; *Report of the Census of Production for 1954,* Industry B, Table 5.
6. *Report of the Departmental Committee on Night Baking,* Cmd. 5525, 1937, para. 46; Maunder, op. cit., pp.21-7.
7. R. Evely & I.M.D. Little, *Concentration in British Industry,* Cambridge, 1960, p.254. An important enabling factor was the development of road transport after 1920 which brought the plant baker to the master baker's doorstep. For a summary of technical developments in the bakery industry see J.B. Jefferys, *Retail Trading in Britain 1850-1950,* Cambridge, 1954, pp.211-13.
8. Ibid., Ch.VII.
9. Evely & Little, op. cit., pp.257-8.
10. Maunder, op. cit., p.111.
11. I am grateful to a number of master bakers in the Reading and Newbury areas of Berkshire for this and other information.
12. For a detailed survey of changes in the grocery and bread and flour confectionery trades up to 1950, see Jefferys, op. cit., Ch. V, VII.
13. *Census of Distribution,* 1961, Pt. 1, Establishment Table 3, 9, 14, Organisation Table 8.
14. H. Rothman & D. Radford, 'Selling the staff of life', *New Scientist,* 22 August 1974, pp.458-9.
15. NFS, 1958, 1970; Jefferys, op. cit., p.218. In the north of England and in Scotland the proportion of wrapped bread sold by multiple shop bakers was over 75 per cent in the late thirties. ibid., p.218. In 1970, c.70% of white bread was bought wrapped, NFS, 1970.
16. Collins, loc. cit.; NFS, 1970.

17. W. Tibbles, *Foods,* 1912, p.417.
18. The Ryvita company which was founded by the Campbell Garrett family was subsequently taken over by Rowntree Ltd. and from them by Associated British Foods. The Birmingham bakery was bombed out in World War Two and a new central bakery opened at Poole, Dorset, in 1949. Private communication, Ryvita Company Ltd.
19. For a comprehensive summary of the brown and white bread controversy see R. McCance & E. Widdowson, *Brown Breads and White,* 1956.
20. The foregoing information about the history of Hovis Limited has been kindly supplied by the firm of Rank Hovis McDougall Ltd. This is not intended as a comprehensive review of the activities of the firm but is concerned mainly with advertising and promotion. The more general history is summarised in *The Hovis Jubilee: a Brief Record of the Company's History between 1898-1948,* (privately printed, London, 1948).
21. H.V. Edwards, 'Flour milling', in M.P. Fogarty (ed.), *Further Studies in Industrial Organisation,* 1948, p.46.
22. W. Crawford & H. Broadley, *The Peoples' Food,* 1938, pp.168-9.
23. NFS, 1950-1972.
24. The following survey of the historical development of the American breakfast cereals industry is based on Gerald Carson, *Cornflake Crusade,* 1959, and on information provided by the Kellogg Co., Battle Creek, Michigan, USA. The basic manufacturing techniques are explained in J.S. Remington, 'Breakfast cereal foods', *Food Manufacture,* Sept. 1935, pp.305-19, and more recent developments (in the USA) in *Studies of Organization and Competition in Grocery Manufacturing,* Nat. Committee on Food Marketing, Study No. 6, 1966, Ch. 9.
25. The transition from a health food with a limited appeal to a utility food with a popular appeal is perhaps the most important aspect of the historical development of breakfast cereals. Indicative of the new status of breakfast cereals were changes in nomenclature – 'Post Toasties' for 'Elijah's Manna', and the Kellogg Co. for the Sanitas Nut Food Company. Most breakfast cereals were originally marketed as 'natural', 'biologic' or, in the case of Grape Nuts, 'brain' foods. Post was a multi-millionaire by 1911 but W.K. Kellogg was the more successful entrepreneur; he had little sympathy with health reform and in 1911 bought out J.H. Kellogg's interest in the Battle Creek Toasted Corn Flake Co.
26. *Studies of Organization and Competition in Grocery Manufacturing,* op. cit. *The Structure of Food Manufacturing,* National Committee on Food Marketing, Technical Study No. 8, 1966, pp.11-13.
27. Tibbles, op. cit., p.443ff.
28. Private communication: Quaker Oats Ltd.
29. *Grocer,* 4 July 1970.
30. *A Report on the Supply of Ready-cooked Breakfast Cereal Foods,* Monopolies Commission, 1973, p.3.
31. Tibbles, op. cit., p.443ff.
32. Private communication: Quaker Oats Ltd.
33. 'The manufacture of shredded wheat', *Food Manufacture,* 1, No. 2 (1927), pp.44-6; *Breakfast Cereals,* Monopolies Commission report, op. cit., p.4.
34. ibid., p.4.
35. Private communication: Mr. Roy Richards, marketing director, Weetabix Ltd., who gave me a valuable first insight into the workings of the breakfast cereals industry in the post-war period.
36. Private communication: Quaker Oats Ltd. I have been unable, however, to locate the original survey.
37. Private communication: Quaker Oats Ltd; *Breakfast Cereals,* Monopolies

Commission report, op. cit., p.7.
38. ibid., p.5
39. Stone & Rowe, op. cit., p.23.
40. *Breakfast Cereals,* Monopolies Commission report, op. cit., p.7.
41. ibid., p.4.
42. NFS, 1942-50. The wartime estimates are crude and probably inaccurate as consumption has been derived from unit price and expenditure data.
43. NFS, 1950-70.
44. NFS, 1950-70. In 1968 total breakfast cereal sales were estimated at £46m, of which RTE comprised £40m, traditional porridge £4m and instant cereals £2m. *Grocer,* 18 Jan. 1969. Porridge sales were claimed to have fallen by 27% in Scotland between 1965 and 1969. *Grocer,* 25 April 1970.
45. *Breakfast Cereals,* Monopolies Commission report, op. cit., p.4; NFS (including summary pre-war data 1940-72).
46. e.g. Crawford & Broadley, op. cit.; J.B. Orr, *Food, Health and Income,* 1936; *Family Diet and Health in Pre-war Britain,* Carnegie Trust, Dunfermline, 1955.
47. B.S. Rowntree, *Poverty and Progress,* 1941, p.189.
48. Collins, loc. cit.; Crawford & Broadley, op. cit., p.39ff. In the USA oatmeal was first popularised as a breakfast food by a German immigrant, Ferdinand Schumacher, of Ohio, and the first advertisement appeared in a local newspaper in 1870.
49. ibid., pp.39ff, 166ff; NFS, 1970.
50. Crawford & Broadley, op. cit., p.39ff; G.C. Warren (ed.), *The Foods We Eat,* 1958, p.23ff; *Grocer,* 10 July 1965; *Grocer,* 8 July 1967.
51. *Grocer,* 23 April 1921; 29 April 1922. The early twenties marked the beginnings of really intensive competition between porridge and RTE cereals. Vernons awarded prizes to shopkeepers for novel and attractive solo window displays and emphasised the ways in which their containers could be used for model-making — Tower Bridge, crockery sets, etc. Scotts of Colinton, Midlothian, makers of 'the food of a mighty race', distributed booklets and brochures, *Grocer,* 8 Oct. 1921, 18 Feb. 1922.
52. e.g. Quaker Instant Porridge, Scott-Cerebos 'Flying Start', Lyons' 'Ready Brek'.
53. *Breakfast Cereals,* Monopolies Commission report, op. cit., p.5. Kellogg spent 13% in 1930-32, 20% in 1933, 27.7% in 1935 and 18.2% in 1939.
54. N. Kaldor & R. Silverman, *A Statistical Analysis of Advertising Expenditure and of the Revenue of the Press,* Cambridge, 1948, p.144; breakfast cereal ratios were exceeded by those of malted health foods (41%) and beef extracts and essences (22%), ibid., p.144.
55. F.P. Bishop, *The Economics of Advertising,* 1944, pp.83, 87.
56. The crucial role of advertising in the growth of the modern food industry is a subject all by itself. The emphases were successively those of (a) posters and billboards, (b) national press, (c) television. Newspapers allowed display ads only after 1870 and this became a main source of revenue for national newspapers and popular magazines betweens the wars. Between 1910 and 1930 display advert space in eight London dailies more than doubled, and in four London dailies advertising volume (space *x* circulation) rose tenfold.
(F.W. Taylor, *The Economics of Advertising,* 1934, p.212ff). In 1930 one leading RTE firm spent 35% of its advertising appropriation in newspapers and magazines, 10% on posters and 35% on dealer aids: ibid., p.228. For general reading see Taylor, op.cit., Bishop, op. cit., D. & G. Hindley, *Advertising in Victorian England, 1837-1901,* 1972; P. Hadley, *The History of Bovril Advertising,* 1974.
57. Consumer research shows that in 1963 over 70% of households served RTE

cereals, with the greatest concentration in houses with young children. The trade recognises two types of brands, 'basic' and 'switch'. Some cereals (e.g. Corn Flakes, Shredded Wheat and Weetabix) were 'family' cereals, others like All Bran and Special K 'health' cereals, and the majority 'children's' cereals. Advertising techniques reflected these differences. *Retail Business Special Report,* 1964, pp.17ff.

58. Private communication: Quaker Oats Ltd; *Breakfast Cereals,* Monopolies Commission report, op. cit., p.7; *The Buying Habits of Daily Herald Readers,* 4th ser., No. 3, 1956, pp.5-8. Force Wheat Flakes ceased to be imported after 1939 but were reintroduced, on a limited scale, in 1970.
59. ibid., p.19; 'When U.S. products fail', *Marketing,* May 1970, pp.26-9.
60. R.D. Buzzell & R.E.M. Nourse, *Product Innovation, the Product Life Cycle and Competitive Behaviour in Selected Food Processing Industries 1947-64,* A.D. Little Inc., Cambridge, Mass. 1966.
61. Figures for the UK are not available but in the USA it was estimated that in 1967 43 per cent of 'prepared breakfast foods' were new (i.e. post-1957) products. *Food Marketing and Economic Growth,* OECD, Paris, 1970, pp.36-7.
62. Bishop, op. cit., p.87.
63. *Breakfast Cereals,* Monopolies Commission report, op. cit., p.13; Maunder, op. cit., p.91.
64. Quoted Taylor, op. cit., p.47.

4 THE DEVELOPMENT OF THE MEAT INDUSTRY
E.F. WILLIAMS

Meat as Food

From a scientific point of view our knowledge of meat as an item of diet with regard to nutrition, biochemistry, histology, structure and quality is barely fifty years old. Furthermore, it is only about two hundred years since there was a determined effort to breed and feed animals specifically for the production of good quality meat. Prior to this, although domestication of several species of animals can be traced back for five to seven thousand years, i.e. about the time of some form of settled agriculture, there are indications to suggest that man has since the dawn of history eaten the flesh of animals (and sometimes man) whenever possible. As archaeological records show that man has consumed a wide variety of animals for food, many of which are now extinct, I should commence by defining what today is considered to be meat. In the simplest terms, meat may be defined as the flesh of animals commonly used as food,[1] although in practice this definition has been widened to include organs such as the heart, liver, kidney, brains and other edible parts, for example, intestines used in the manufacture of sausage.

Although there are some three thousand mammalian species, very few may be described as commonly used for food and in the United Kingdom the bulk of meat consumed is derived from cattle, sheep, pigs, poultry and game. In other parts of the world, however, meat derived from horse, goat and deer is regularly consumed and, in fact, a number of other species are used for meat depending on availability and local custom. Thus, for example, the camel, seal, polar bear, kangaroo and the whale form an important part of the diet of certain communities. It would appear that from the dawn of history, man in his struggle for survival has had to match his powers against two- and four-legged animals and when he was successful he ate as much of his opponent as possible.[2]

It was this practice of eating meat to the full whenever it was available which was noted by Hippocrates when he contended that 'perhaps in those days man suffered terribly from their indigestible and animal-like diet, eating raw and uncooked food. . . They suffered as men would suffer now from such a diet, being liable to violent pain and a speedy death.'[3] While vegetarians would no doubt agree with this view, man has always regarded meat as a highly desirable part of the diet and, furthermore, it is an easily digested food and a very efficient source of protein needed for the repair and replacement of tissue in man.

When some form of settled agriculture began to develop, man began to depend increasingly on the cooked flesh of tamed animals and those communities who could not or, for various reasons, would not farm, for example, the Eskimo, the Central African or the Australian Aboriginal, were forced to obtain their meats from fish, marine animals and birds. In those times when food supplies became scarce and hunger became a serious problem, the more dangerous beasts would be attacked, for example, the polar bear, lion and crocodile, and when the occasion arose man would also attack man to provide meat. From the recommendations of recent cannibals, human flesh is known to be tasty to eat and is certainly no less nutritious than other meats. It has been suggested that the number of human beings in existence, particularly in the later stages of man's evolution, from Upper Palaeolithic times onwards, was probably sufficiently large to enable the consumption of human meat to be practicable on more than ceremonial occasions. It is unlikely that the particular qualities of human flesh or severe protein deficiency would have been factors in the evolution of this practice.

It is more probable that the development of flesh-eating began with the need to defend group rights, to hunt and collect from given territories and, therefore, any fatal conflicts resulting from such socio-economic clashes being put to good use. Presumably, when a community is living from day to day on the food resources immediately at hand, it is hardly likely to waste such wholesome meat whether it be friend or enemy. There appears to be little doubt that cannibalism was practised among the early peoples in both the new and the old worlds but, although some of the evidence is not entirely convincing, the discovery in 1929 of the remains of more than forty individuals in the excavations in South-West Peking clearly indicates that originally these had been used for food. There also appears to be strong evidence that Peking man used fire for cooking or roasting meat, and ate the tissues of the now extinct species of bison, horse, deer, bear, sheep, camel and the wild boar. There is also evidence that he cracked bones to extract the marrow and the skulls for brains. However, the meat trade concerned with the consumption of human flesh has completely disappeared and consideration must now be given to the history of those meats other than man, which formed the basis of today's meat trade.

The Origins of Meat Animals

It has been suggested that the ancestors of cattle, sheep and pigs — which today form the main sources of our meat animals — were probably undifferentiated from those of man prior to about sixty million years ago when it is presumed the first mammal appeared on earth.[5] It is possible that by one to two million years ago the species of man, to which we belong, and the wild ancestors of our domesticated animals, i.e. sheep, cattle and pigs, may well have been recognisable. There appear to be some archaeological indications of the hunting of these animals from at least 500,000 BC and there is some evidence — slender as it is — that reindeer were hunted by dogs from the middle of the last ice age, i.e. about 18,000 BC. It was not until the climatic changes arising from the end of this period, i.e. ten to twelve thousand years ago, that conditions favoured the domestication of animals by man, and it is about this time that there appears to be definite evidence that this was so.

It has been suggested by Zeuner[6] that the first stages in the domestication of animals by man involved loose contacts with free breeding. This phase was probably followed by the confinement of animals with breeding in captivity, leading finally to some form of selected breeding, developing breeds with certain desired characteristics, and exterminating the wild ancestors. Domestication was clearly linked with the development of agriculture and, although there is evidence that sheep were domesticated by 7000 BC, control of cattle and pigs did not come about until there was some degree of settled agriculture, i.e. about 5000 BC.

It is interesting to note that the long period of domestication has resulted in a number of changes with regard to the physical characteristics of animals;[7] for example, the size of domesticated animals is usually somewhat smaller than that of their wild ancestors. The colouring alters and there is a tendency for the facial part of the skull to be shorter and additionally the limbs tend to be shorter and thicker. The changes in the structure of the bones has been attributed to the higher plane of nutrition which domestication permits. It has been suggested that many of the domesticated characteristics are, in fact, juvenile ones persisting to the adult stage.[8] Thus, the present Middle White pig is somewhat smaller than the wild pig, its skull is more juvenile and lacking the pointed features of the wild boar, its legs are shorter and the skin lacks hair and pigment.

Domesticated sheep appear to have originated in Western Asia and there is evidence that they were domesticated with the aid of dogs long before there was any form of settled agriculture. From archaeological friezes it is apparent that by 3500—3000 BC several breeds of domestic sheep were well established in Mesopotamia and Egypt. The domestication of sheep appears to be associated with the development of a longer tail, the horns tend to rise less steeply and the wool is much less pigmented as compared with the wild breeds. Little attempt appears to have been made to improve the characteristics of sheep with regard to meat and wool production until the marked changes in agriculture in the early eighteenth century.

Currently in the UK there are about forty breeds of improved sheep[9] which may be roughly divided into three main classes, namely the hill breeds, long wool breeds and the down breeds. There are today some twenty hill breeds in the UK of which the Scotch Blackface, Cheviot, Welsh Mountain, Shetland, Dartmore and the Swaledale are representative. Of the long wool breeds, probably the best known are the Romney Marsh, Lincoln, Cotswold, South Devon, and the Leicester. There are now more than ten down breeds of which the Southdown, Dorset Down, Suffolk, Shropshire Down and the Hampshire are probably the best known. The present improved breeds, such as the Suffolk, tend to give a greater carcase yield than the semi-wild breeds, such as the Shetland, largely because of their increased fatness. Those breeds which are early maturing such as the Southdown, have a higher proportion of fat than the later maturing breeds such as the Lincoln and the Welsh.

With regard to cattle there was apparently little or no domestication until the establishment of some form of settled agriculture about 5000 BC and according to Zeuner, domesticated hump-backed cattle existed in Mesopotamia by 4500 BC and the large horned cattle of Egypt by about 4000 BC.

The Development of Carcase Meat Animals

The major development of many breeds of cattle for meat did not come about until the marked changes in agriculture in the UK in the early part of the eighteenth century when Bakewell initiated improvements by the introduction of in-breeding, the use of proven sires and the practice of selection and culling. In the UK prior to this time, cattle had been used primarily for draught purposes or for milk.

The changes initiated by Bakewell appear to be the first real attempt to produce cattle for meat, which would fatten quickly when the skeletal growth was complete. This has resulted in a trend towards smaller and leaner animals which were slaughtered at a much earlier age, examples of which are the Aberdeen Angus, the Hereford and some of the North Devon breeds. For reasons which will be discussed later, there is a possibility that this trend towards smaller animals may be arrested and in fact reversed. Since the early developments by Bakewell and the more recent knowledge of the effects of a high plane of nutrition, there has been a growing realisation that the full breed potentialities will not be fully developed without adequate food given at the right time in the growth pattern of the animal.

According to Gerrard[10] the dairy and beef Shorthorns are the predominant breed in terms of numbers in the UK but the Aberdeen Angus is regarded by the trade as the premier breed for the best quality meat. The Angus, Hereford and North Devon conform to the general view today that a beef animal should be well covered with flesh, blocky and compact, thus reducing the proportion of bone. Muscle development is marked over the hindquarters, along the back and down the legs.

The beef breeds in the UK consist largely of the Aberdeen Angus, Hereford, West Highland, Devon and Galloway, all of which give a high proportion of cuts which are in great demand and all of which, with suitable management, yield meat which is tender and succulent. The predominant dairy types are the Ayrshire, Friesian, Jersey, Guernsey and the Kerry and although these breeds were developed for milk production, a considerable quantity of beef is derived from this source.

It was not until about 150 years ago that European pigs began to change as they were crossed with imported Chinese breeds. The long-snouted razor-backed animal with a sloping back and little development of the hindquarter gave way to the relatively short round back of uniform height and well-developed hindquarters but over fat. This type of breed has been further improved to give a longer animal, for example, the Landrace, light in the forequarter, with a small head, but heavy in the hindquarter. Until quite recently in the UK the Middle White and the Berkshire were regarded as the most useful pigs for pork production, the Large White, Essex, Large Black and the Gloucester for bacon and pork, and the Welsh, Landrace and Tamworth for bacon production. However, with the changes in retailing, butchery methods and considerable changes in curing methods, the Large White crossed with the Landrace, and pure Landrace probably form the bulk of pigs grown in the UK.

The improvement in pigs has not been continuous in one direction but has been related to changing requirements at different periods. In line with the improvements in cattle, the first and subsequent breeds to be brought to a high standard originated in England. For example, the Berkshire crossed with the Western County breed in the USA helped to establish the Poland China breed over a century ago and this formed the basis for American pork production. Unlike cattle, it is possible to change the types within a short time and this was well demonstrated when the Poland China was changed from a heavy round-backed lard-type pig to a long lean bacon pig within twelve years. However, the changes in types have not always been to our advantage and I hope to demonstrate this point later.

Trade in Meat

So far mention has only been made of changes involved in the production of carcase meat but there is much evidence that by the early Roman period a considerable meat trade existed and meat shops resembling the small butchers' shops of today existed and were apparently conducted in a sanitary manner. Furthermore the curing and salting of hams and the production of a range of cured and smoked sausage was well established and a wide range of herbs and spices was used in the products. According to Jensen[11] the ancient Roman butchers and meat chefs prepared and used cracklings, bacon, tenderloin, salt pork bellies and all kinds of steaks and hams. They apparently were well-versed in the techniques of boning beef, lamb, veal and pigs and also dealt in wholesale and retail cuts much like those of today. Yet, as mentioned before, despite the continuing and increasing demand for meat and the very substantial increase in animal numbers throughout the world there is little evidence that any attempt was made either by breeding or selection to obtain meat from animals bred for the purpose.

With the spread of Roman knowledge in meat handling and processing to Europe the trade began to develop and improve, until by about 1000 AD London had numerous abattoirs to supply the growing population, and although it is not known whether they were effective there were regulations in force for butchering and handling of meat. Guilds of butchers were in existence in William the Conqueror's reign (1080) and have remained through English history up to the present day.

Although there is evidence to suggest that man utilised animals as a source of food since the dawn of history, it was not until the profound changes in agriculture in the UK during the eighteenth century that the entire concept of raising animals specifically for meat began to change. Prior to that time, there was no systematic feeding of animals, which is hardly surprising as knowledge of nutrition is quite recent; furthermore there was no knowledge of genetics. The major changes in agriculture, which commenced about 1750, gave increased acreages of wheat, turnips, oil cake, swedes and potatoes and this in turn provided a higher standard of nutrition for the animals during the winter and early spring. In scarcely more than a century farming methods advanced from a state little less primitive than that of the Middle Ages into something not greatly inferior to those in use today. This, in turn, resulted in better-quality meat animals and a more uniform pattern of slaughtering throughout the year, but it was the advent of the industrial revolution which brought about more rapid changes in the meat industry than at any time in history.

Prior to this, animals were slaughtered on farms or the local abattoir and the meat was largely consumed locally but as the demand for industrial labour increased, more and more people moved into the towns and cities and became entirely dependent on the food supplied or manufactured by others. For example, by 1850 there were over 2.5 million people in London, all of whom had to be fed. This resulted in the building of large abattoirs in the city centres to provide meat for the masses and without the advantage of refrigeration it was necessary to move large numbers of animals to the markets and *abattoirs* in the cities where the population was beginning to concentrate. Cattle, sheep and pigs were, therefore, driven on the hoof from the growing areas, sometimes for considerable distances, to be slaughtered in the major towns and cities. By 1850 the total production of meat, i.e. beef, pork and mutton, in the UK had risen to about 900,000 tons providing about 72 lbs. per head per year. This was supplemented by importing animals to give a further 44,000 tons making a total of about 75 lbs. per head of population yearly. In the next thirty years the total tonnage had risen to about 1.25 million, giving a *per capita* consumption of about 110 lbs., and it stayed at that level until refrigeration was established.

Today we accept the refrigeration of meat as a normal method of preservation — what may not be appreciated is that it was not until 1880 that the first successful shipment of beef took place. Its development was, of course, one of the direct results of the industrial revolution when demands for meat called for the discovery of some means for the safe delivery of those supplies. The uneasiness concerning meat supplies in England became very marked by the middle of the nineteenth century and the growth of the manufacturing industries made it clear that the UK must be an increasingly important meat consumer. Manufacturing, particularly in the heavy industries, demanded energetic flesh-fed men, but meat supplies and prices were worse than they had been for many years. It was natural, therefore, that attention should be drawn to the possibility of shipping meat in a frozen condition from Australia or America where supplies were both plentiful and cheap. No serious development along these lines could take place until a means of providing cheap ice was available or until a refrigeration plant had been invented. It was at this period when attention was drawn to an idea by a French engineer who stated that under suitable conditions compressed ammonia gas could be used as a refrigerant but it was some thirty years before the idea was developed and used for the first shipment of refrigerated meat from South America. The voyage to Rouen in France took over three months, but despite this length of time at least part of the cargo was still edible. In February 1880, the s.s. Strathleven arrived in London with 40 tons of refrigerated beef and mutton all of which was in good condition, at least by the prevailing standards. It was sold on Smithfield market for an average of 5½*d.* per lb., i.e. slightly more expensive than today, allowing for the change in values.

Because of the growing demand for meat, the total stocks of animals in the UK continued to increase so that between 1850 and 1880 they had risen from 41 million to 46 million and it is interesting to note that during the same thirty years the population of the UK had also grown from about 27 million to 34 million. By the middle of the nineteenth century, manufactured meat products of every variety and every level of quality were marketed in all major towns and cities and consumed by the ever-increasing number of people migrating from the rural areas. At the same time, canned meats were beginning to appear and yet, despite a wider variety of foods and an allegedly high consumption of meat, there was hardly a time in history when the standard of health and nutrition was lower, and it was well into the twentieth century before the health and the nutritional status of the working population began to improve.

It was during the latter part of the seventeenth century that the American so-called meat packing industry began to develop. According to Schweigert[12] it was the New England farmers who began to pack in salt not only pork and beef but also venison and bear meat and this started what is now a huge meat manufacturing industry. Before the end of the century live animals were being driven in considerable numbers and over fairly long distances to be killed and salted down. By the mid-nineteenth century large packing houses were built in Chicago, Buffalo and Cincinatti — it was the latter town that according to Schweigert became known as Porkopolis — where a system was perfected of packing 15 bushels of maize into a hog and then packing the carcase into a barrel with salt. Rapid developments in the fields of engineering and technology then opened the way for considerable expansion and mechanisation of the industry and this led to the line system where the entire operation of slaughtering, dressing, butchering, curing and canning was a continuous conveyorised process.

By the early 1900s, when refrigeration was proving its value, a very substantial industry had developed both in America and the United Kingdom largely through a gradual evolution of traditional processing, production and distribution procedures, but little thought appears to have been given to the welfare of the animal about to be slaughtered. The rapid advance in technology and the need for efficiency clearly outstripped humanitarian principles. For example, the method of killing pigs in an American packing house consisted of shackling the hind leg of the animal to a horizontal moving track, thus forcibily dragging it backwards until the shackle was automatically transferred to a large wheel. On this the pigs were elevated to the floor above where their throats were cut without any form of anaesthetic. By improving efficiency, killing rates have increased from about 60–100 in a non-mechanised abattoir to about 1,200 an hour in a modern plant but this, in turn, has raised a number of problems with regard to loss of meat quality caused primarily by pre-slaughter stress in the animal. Similarly, beef animals were driven in to slaughter but because of the difficulty, i.e. size and strength of the animal, they were rendered (sometimes) unconsicous by a 'knocker'. This gentleman was armed with an instrument consisting of a hammer head attached to a long handle and it was his task to aim a blow at the forehead of the animal. Unfortunately, the animal could not be relied upon to remain stationary and undue suffering was caused. This method has now been largely replaced by the captive bolt or electric stunning, both of which are more humane and efficient although it is known that these methods cause defects in meat quality.

Meat production in the USA was largely developed by seven companies but it was Swifts who, by the early part of the twentieth century, had seven large packing houses capable of transforming into meat about 11,000 cattle, 16,000 sheep and 35,000 pigs in one day. By 1930 meat production had reached 8 million tons rising to over 13 million tons in 1960. During the same period the *per capita* consumption of meat rose from about 130 lbs. in 1930 to 150 lbs. in 1960 and the figure for 1973 was about 190 lbs.

In the development of this huge industry, it was apparently overlooked that certain diseases in animals could be transmitted to man, and any animal, provided it could walk into the abattoir, was fairly certain to end up as carcase meat or a meat product. There is evidence that some form of meat hygiene began with the earliest civilisations of the Mediterranean area. For instance, in ancient Egypt the pig was regarded as unclean and the cow sacred and, therefore, banned as a source of meat. The slaughtering of oxen, geese and goats, the staple meats, and also the slaughtering of the ibex and gazelle, was governed by elaborate rules. It is probable that the rules were linked to religious taboos as much as to sanitation. The Israelites adopted these principles about 2000 BC but also prohibited the use of blood for food and, therefore, demanded complete bleeding of the animal; in addition, a number of rules concerning hand washing and personal hygiene were introduced. These Mosaic Laws, which are still observed by Orthodox Jews and Mohammedans, form the basis for our present rules of hygiene.

Since the dawn of history there has been a demand for the flesh of animals for food but there has been a recognition that meat can also be the cause of ill-health due to the presence of pathogenic organisms within the meat or from subsequent contamination. The basic purpose of meat hygiene is to prevent spoilage and, as far as possible, to prevent access by pathogenic organisms. Similarly, the epidemiology of meat-borne diseases is mainly concerned with the nature, source and method of spread and growth of these organisms. The early Roman writers suggested that there were similarities between diseases in man and in animals but in the Middle Ages, without our present knowledge of bacteriology, meat inspection was almost non-existent and where carried out was met with heavy opposition. There is some evidence that meat inspection was practised in France as early as 1162 and in Germany inspection of pigs became allegedly compulsory in 1385. In

England, the passing of the Urban Sanitary Act in 1388 — at least theoretically — provided for some form of examination of carcase meat. It was not, however, until the introduction of the Food & Drugs Act of 1938 that any real attempt was made to inspect meat. In North America, only rudimentary meat inspection was carried out in a few cities before 1884 when the Federal Bureau of the Animal Industry was formed. This was re-established under the Food & Drugs Act of 1906. By 1949, only one-third of the animals slaughtered was inspected and even today not all the animals slaughtered in the USA are fully inspected. Thus, although there have been great strides and rapid progress in meat technology, particularly in the last hundred years, the progress in meat hygiene and meat inspection has been almost painfully slow.

Scientific Breeding

I have previously mentioned that from the early eighteenth century to the early twentieth century there were profound changes in agriculture and animal husbandry which resulted in considerable improvement and development of domestic animals specifically for meat production. Most of these changes were brought about by farmers and breed societies and it was not until quite recently that science began to take an active part. Thus, in the last fifty to seventy years a considerable effort has gone into the rearing and feeding of cattle, sheep and pigs. Changes in animal husbandry and the efforts of geneticists and nutritionists have resulted in breeds of meat animals which apparently have most of the characteristics that are now required, i.e. the ratio of meat to bone is high, the animals are well muscled — particularly in the most desirable part — they grow rapidly and produce good quality meat with a high ratio of lean to fat. In order to achieve these results, extensive use has been made of progeny testing based on carcase measurements and this has been recognised as an efficient way of hastening the evolution of animals having those body proportions most desirable for the consumer.

Artificial insemination has afforded the means of vastly increasing the number of progeny which can be sired by a given animal having the desired characteristics. The geneticists and physiologists are striving to produce multiple births in sheep and cattle and the nutritionists, in collaboration with the manufacturers of animal feed, have developed means of inducing more rapid growth. Growth-promoting additives, hormones and antibiotics have all been used in an attempt to produce more meat in a shorter time. These developments, coupled in some instances with the doubtful practice of confining animals during the growing period with little or no room for movement, have resulted in considerable opposition in some quarters.

Rachel Carsons, in the early 1960s, strongly criticised American beef production by referring to the practice of artificial insemination, the use of hormones, antibiotics and tranquillisers, radioactive fall-out on the pasturage and inhumane methods of slaughter. Despite criticism, the fact remains that there have been considerable improvements in food conversion, rate of growth and animal health. However, it should be noted that improving growth rates, food conversion efficiency and the production of more lean meat in an animal has led to the appearance of certain defects in the quality of the meat, particularly in pigs. This was apparent in the development of the Danish Landrace and the Pietran-type pigs, and to some extent in beef, in which a proportion of the animals become stress-prone and produce what is known as PSE (pale, soft and exudative) meat, a defect which often causes problems associated with curing.

Despite the rapid advances made in the quality and breeds of animals for meat, it is interesting to note that meat science, i.e. the study of the conversion of the living animal into meat and its subsequent handling, did not commence until just before 1930. It was only then that scientists began to study all aspects of the procedures and mechanisms concerned with converting the living animal into meat. There was little or no scientifically based knowledge concerned with the technology or preservation of meat and certainly no knowledge of the biochemical changes which occur when a living muscle is converted into meat. Nevertheless, during the past fifty years a considerable volume of scientific knowledge has accumulated. Basic studies have unravelled many of the biochemical changes which occur during *rigor mortis;* the causes of toughness or tenderness in meat are now fairly well understood and the effects of stress on the living animal and its relation to meat quality are slowly being unravelled.

Meat microbiology and methods of maintaining a high standard of hygiene are no longer shrouded in mystery, the technology of refrigeration has not only helped in the field of hygiene but has enabled highly perishable carcase meat to be handled, shipped and displayed for sale without loss of quality. Overall there is now a very healthy background of scientific knowledge concerned with all aspects of meat from the living animal to the consumer's plate and, therefore, it would be expected that the meat industry would take full advantage of science to improve methods and efficiency. Unfortunately this is not so and in many cases methods used for the handling and slaughtering of animals have hardly changed for several hundred years.

The reason may be due to the fact that the meat industry, which is highly fragmented, is somewhat conservative and old ideas die hard. This situation is changing. In 1961, for example, there were approximately 42,000 butchers' shops in the UK, but by 1971 there were only about 34,000 and it is probable that in 1974 the number will be only about 30,000. This trend is being accelerated by the large multiples who are now taking an increasing share in the meat trade.

Additionally, the very small abattoirs are disappearing and a larger proportion of animals are being killed in fewer places.

What will be the effect on the industry? If the trend continues the bulk of meat handled in the UK will be in the hands of a very few large companies who will probably control — both scientifically and technologically — all operations from the living animal to the consumer. This should lead to very considerable improvements in live animal handling, *ante* and *post-mortem* inspection, slaughter methods, meat hygiene, transportation and temperature control at all stages including display for sale. Already there are some companies who have made very substantial progress in all fields of meat handling; others will follow if and when they realise the advantages of using the scientific knowledge which is available. The meat industry today in the UK is by no means small. The retail value of meat is approximately £2,500 million to which must be added about £100 million for the catering trade; and if wastage is to be reduced and efficiency improved full use must be made of current scientific knowledge.

What is likely to be the situation with regard to meat and meat products in the future? The increasing pressure of world population and the need to raise living standards have made the production of more and better meat, more effective preservation, and the elimination of waste, important issues. It is probable that the demand for animal protein in the UK will have increased by over 300 per cent by the year 2000 compared with 1960. In the less developed countries, however, the consumption of meat can be as low as 14 lbs. per head per year, and clearly to raise this by even a small amount would require a very considerable increase in the animal population, even assuming that the human population remained at its present level. The current world population is approximately 3,000 millions and it is postulated that the doubling time is about thirty years; in other words, by the end of the century the global population might be about 6—7,000 millions. In the last few years in the UK the rate of growth has been reduced and the current forecast suggests that we are unlikely to reach the levels indicated in earlier reports. Nevertheless, it is forecast that the UK population could be about 60 millions by the end of the century and, therefore, the demand for meat and meat products must inevitably increase quite considerably.

How is this to be met? Several possibilities exist with regard to cattle for beef production, for example, by a higher incidence of twin births, the further development of dual purpose animals for both beef and milk, and the utilisation of some of the larger breeds. The recent world shortage of beef has emphasised the need to increase the weight of lean meat derived from each calf, yet modern methods of intensive production tend to reduce not only the age at which the animal is slaughtered but also the slaughter-weight. One of the problems, therefore, is how to raise cattle intensively but to a much higher weight at slaughter than is currently generally accepted and at the same time maintain or improve quality. The recent change in government policy with regard to the importation of some of the larger breeds from Europe has now brought many of these breeds under scrutiny. The European practice of raising bulls, which are leaner and more efficient food converters when compared with the steer, coupled with the use of the larger breeds, could be an interesting development. For example, the Italian Chianina breed when fully grown stands at about 6 ft. at the shoulder and weighs up to 4,000 lbs. Thus, commercially it should be possible to produce animals weighing about 2,000 lbs. at the age of about two years with a lean carcase weighing approximately half a ton. A further increase in animal protein might well be obtained by an extension of the present restricted list of animals commonly used as a source of meat. Magnus Pyke[13] has drawn attention to the large areas of the African continent which appear to be basically unsuitable to traditional farming from which substantial quantities of meat could be harvested. Many of these wild species produce meat at least as efficiently as cattle bred for the purpose.

There is still much to be done to increase the tonnage of meat throughout the world and time is not on our side. In the meantime, other sources of protein are being developed and non-meat meat products derived from vegetable protein are already commercially viable and are now beginning to reach the consumer. The USA, which is the largest producer of soya bean, was the first to utilise the extracted protein and by extrusion or spinning developed a wide range of food products. Similar processes have also been developed in the UK and the spun protein which on suitable treatment can resemble meat is now being incorporated into meat products, for example, in chopped meat pies. Although the price of meat in the UK could possibly come down because of increased supplies, it is unlikely that production will ever keep pace with the increase in purchasing power of the population. Thus plant proteins could well have a future as there may not be enough high quality protein available. Additionally, proteins from yeasts, various types of micro-organisms from petroleum oil and from natural gas are being increasingly studied. It might well be that in the future in order to obtain sufficient quantities of animal protein it may be necessary to sacrifice, at least to some extent, the current concept of quality but clearly if it is a matter of slightly lower quality beef or no beef or too little beef, we may have no choice.

Notes

1. R.A. Lawrie, *Meat Science,* Pergamon, 1974.
2. C.E. Dolman, *Meat Hygiene,* FAO Monograph 33, 1967.
3. J. Chadwick and W.N. Mann, *The Medical Works of Hippocrates,* Oxford, 1950.
4. L.B. Jensen, *Man's Foods,* Garrard, 1953.
5. Lawrie, op. cit.
6. F.E. Zeuner, *A History of Domesticated Animals,* Hutchinson, 1963.
7. Lawrie, op. cit.
8. J. Hammond, *Pig Breeders' Annual,* National Pig Breeders' Association, 1933.
9. F. Gerrard, *Meat Technology,* Hill, 1951.
10. Gerrard, op. cit.
11. L.B. Jensen, *Microbiology of Meats,* Garrard, 1954.
12. B.S. Schweigert, and H.A. Armstrong, *The Science of Meat and Meat Products,* Freeman, San Francisco, 1960.
13. M. Pyke, *Man and Food,* World University Library, 1960.

5 THE GROWTH OF THE SUGAR TRADE AND REFINING INDUSTRY

G.N. JOHNSTONE

The sugar supply of the world today comes roughly 55 per cent from cane and 45 per cent from sugar beet, yet the history of sugar is — until about 1800 — entirely the story of sugar cane. It is in the last 150 years or so only that beet has developed, until today it provides nearly half the world's supply.

The origin of the use of sugar as we know it is veiled in antiquity, but it is possible that man acquired his sweet tooth through the acquaintance of honey. Little enough is known about the beginning of sugar cane, although there is little doubt that it grew in the islands of the Pacific. A very early reference to it can be found in Hindu literature about 500 BC, but it was Nearchus, an admiral of Alexander the Great, who gives us the first definite knowledge of sugar cane cultivation. In 300 BC, when on a voyage to India, he reported that he saw 'reeds that produced honey although there were no bees'. The spread of sugar cane was a slow process. By 600 AD it had reached the Mediterranean countries. Here, owing to its rarity and cost, sugar became the monopoly of the wealthy. The industry centred on Venice, the great trading city of the time, and here it was to remain for the next six hundred years.

In the fifteenth century, sugar made rapid progress westwards. The great Spanish and Portuguese explorers took the cane to Madeira, the Canary Islands, Cape Verde Islands, North Africa and West Africa. It was on his second voyage in 1493 that Columbus took the plant to the new world, establishing it on the island of San Domingo. In this way were started the great West Indian sugar plantations. The spread of sugar eastwards was less rapid, and it was not until 1788 that cane was introduced to Australia, where nowadays along the eastern coastal region in Queensland is a large and flourishing industry.

Refining

It may be appropriate at this point to describe briefly the process used in those days, which, although coming from the Venetian industry, is broadly representative. Sugar juice was expressed or crushed from short sections of cut cane, and this liquor — a dirty, impure fluid — was fed into a clarifying pan. The clarifying pan was filled two-thirds with lime water and one-third with sugar, thus obtaining a melt of equal parts of sugar and water. To this was added a clearing medium of white of egg or of fresh bullock's blood. (Monceau, a French refiner, was of the opinion that blood was the better clarifier. He had tried isinglass, but without good effect.) As soon as the scums had risen to the surface, the fire was drawn and after an interval of a quarter of an hour, the scum was scraped off. The process was repeated until a bright and clear liquor was obtained. When considered satisfactory, the liquor was strained through a blanket, whereafter it was ladled out into the boiling pans.

In boiling conditions the liquor swelled and was controlled by the addition of some butter and by rapid stirring. The boiling took about three-quarters of an hour and the correct moment at which to strike was determined by the sugar master, who removed some material with a proof stick and tested it between finger and thumb, drawing out a thread of material with the thumb below. After the cooling vessel was filled, it was stirred to break up the crust which formed on the surface, then the material was transferred to clay cone-shaped moulds, the narrow end of which was pierced with a hole. After drainage for several days, the sugar loaf was knocked out of its mould and put in a warm, drying area for a week or more. The whole process took as long as a month.

Trade

At the end of the Middle Ages, the knowledge of refining processes, long held in secret, gradually drifted northwards and westwards into Europe. Antwerp replaced Venice as a sugar centre, to be replaced itself eventually by Amsterdam, and by the early seventeenth century refineries were sprouting in Germany and France, in Austria, Holland and Denmark. The first sugar refinery in England was erected in 1544. The English refining industry did not make any substantial progress until the establishment of the raw sugar industry in the West Indies, aided by the Navigation Acts passed in 1660.

Before the British West Indian islands formed the major part of this country's supply, English sugar had come from Holland. The British industry was therefore first located in London where, by the middle of the seventeenth century, there were 50 sugar bakeries. As early as 1620, a refinery had started in Liverpool, and one was in operation in Bristol in 1654. By 1753 there were 120 refineries distributed around the large ports and cities, but with a concentration always around the west coast ports of Liverpool, Bristol and Greenock in Scotland. At this time, raw sugar was costing 34s. a cwt. and refined sold at 62s. a cwt. Such was the cost of the process that these prices showed the refiners a loss.

The British naval blockade of the European coastline during the Napoleonic Wars is credited with being the inducement for Napoleon to establish the French and European beet sugar industry at this time. Indeed, the turn of the nineteenth century, 1800 and the twenty or thirty years thereafter, were significant dates for sugar.

The first twenty years of the nineteenth century saw the dawn of modern sugar refining. Technical innovation and invention were shortly to produce a revolution in manufacturing methods. James Watt had made the steam engine a practical tool. The use of bone charcoal as a de-colourising agent had been put to practical test; the vacuum pan had been invented, thus making the important re-crystallisation stage more rapid and much more economic. Also, in 1837, the centrifugal machine, which was to revolutionise the industry, was invented, although not perfected for practical use until twenty years later. Sir Henry Bessemer, of steel fame, had a hand in this development stage. The suspended centrifugal machine enabled granulated sugar of high quality to be made easily and cheaply so that it quickly became a serious competitor of loaf sugar. And about this time, too, appeared a number of processes for making sugar into slabs which could be cut into cubes or tablets, and now the refined sugar was making its appearance in days, instead of the weeks taken in the loaf process.

The technical changes, the appearance of beet sugar on the scene and the beginning of an era of free trade from about the middle of the nineteenth century — all these factors combined to bring this country to a period when sugar, previously a luxury, was to become much more widely available (see Table I). Thus, up to 1900, there

Table I: *Consumption of Refined Sugar in the UK* (lbs./caput/year)

Period	Consumption	Period	Consumption	Period	Consumption
1700-09	4	1790-99	13.0	1870-74	49.2
1710-19	5	1800-09	18.0	1875-79	53.2
1720-29	8	1810-19	17.0	1880-89	67.9
1730-39	9	1820-29	17.6	1890-99	78.9
1740-49	8	1830-39	17.8	1900-09	84.7
1750-59	8	1840-44	16.4	1910-14	90.8
1760-69	8	1845-49	22.6	1915-19	70.1
1770-79	11	1850-59	30.1	1920-24	69.2
1780-89	12	1860-69	38.7	1924-29	87.8
				1930-37	98.1
				1949-59	99.4
				1959-67	109.5

Source: *The History of Sugar,* Volume II, Noel Deerr, p.532.

was a great increase in refining, but a marked decrease in the number of refineries. In 1900 there were only 13 refineries in Great Britain. Today, 7 refineries are producing four times the quantity that was produced at the beginning of this century.

It is a favourite cry in the sugar industry that sugar has always been a politician's plaything; since sugar is inextricably woven into the agricultural policy of every country in the world where it grows, perhaps it could hardly be otherwise. Certainly, making its appearance as it did, as a luxury or semi-luxury delicacy which later grew and expanded into into an article of wide distribution and common consumption, it was a 'natural' for a tax or duty, and it has continued to illustrate at least two of the classic purposes of a duty, namely, money raising and protection.

Table II: *The Rate of Sugar Duty* (shillings/cwt.)

Year	Foreign	Colonial	Preference
1661	3s. 10d.	1s. 5d.	2s. 5d
1698	7s. 7d.	2s. 10d.	4s. 9d.
1747	15s. 5d.	4s. 10d.	10s. 7d.
1787	27s. 2d.	12s. 4d.	14s. 10d.
1804	59s. 6d.	26s. 6d.	33s. 0d.
1830	66s. 2d.	25s. 2d.	41s. 0d.
1844	66s. 2d. (35s. 8d.)	25s. 0d.	41s. 2d.
1846	63s. 0d. (24s. 6d.)	16s. 4d.	46s. 8d.
1848	21s. 7d.	15s. 2d.	6s. 5d.
1854	14s. 0d.	14s. 0d.	–
1864	11s. 8d.	11s. 8d.	–
1874	NIL	NIL	NIL

The scale of duties given in Table II shows the trend during the period of colonial preference until it was reduced soon after the accession of Queen Victoria, and finally abolished with the beginning of the period of free trade. Duties were assessed until about 1800 on a scale of weights and values, but then the Polariscope was invented, giving an almost instantaneous reading of sugar content, and thereafter scales based on relative purity came into being.

The reintroduction of duties in 1901 to help pay for the Boer War is shown in Table III. Duties rose for the Kaiser's War and again to provide money for Hitler's War.

Sugar Bounties

The European countries early adopted systems of subsidies for their

Table III: *The Rate of Sugar Duty* (shillings/cwt.)

Year	Foreign	Colonial	Preference
1901	4s. 2d.	4s. 2d.	NIL
1908	1s. 10d.	1s. 10d.	NIL
1915	9s. 4d.	9s. 4d.	NIL
1919	25s. 8d.	21s. 5d.	4s. 3d.
1924	11s. 8d.	9s. 9d.	1s. 11d.
1925	11s. 8d.	7s. 5d.	4s. 3d.
1928	11s. 8d.	5s. 10d.	5s. 10d.
1939	23s. 4d.	17s. 6d.	5s. 10d.
1949	11s. 8d.	5s. 10d.	5s. 10d.
1962	6s. 11d.	1s. 1d.	5s. 10d.

exportable surpluses. Between 1850 and 1900 it is estimated that roughly 60 million tons came on the market at prices below the cost of production. Great Britain and the USA were the largest receivers of these surpluses. The effects of these subsidies were, of course, beneficial to the agriculture of the exporting country; elsewhere, however, they had the effect of retarding the development of our own agriculture; causing the failure and close-down of many British refining companies; and lowering the world price of sugar generally.

The trend in world prices in the twentieth century is shown in Table IV. The British market was flooded with cheap raw beet sugar, to the detriment of the cane producers, and a flood of cheap white beet sugar to the detriment of the British refiners. The dramatic fall

Table IV: *UK Retail Sugar Prices*

	Pence per lb.	Possible Factor	1960
1250-1300	15	) x 150 =	175s.
1300-1400	14		
1400-1500	20		150s.
1500-1600	11		42s.
1600-1700	16		27s.
1700-1800	8	) x 20	14s.
1800-1900	4	x 10	3s. 6d.
1920-1930	5.4		2s.
1930-1938	2.4	x 5	1s.
1950-1960	7.2		
1960-to date	9 (approx.)		8½d.

Source: To 1900 – Philip Lyle, *The Sugar Industry,* reprint from the Journal of the Royal Statistical Society.

Amounts Equivalent to 1 lb. Sugar

Period	Cheese	Butter	Eggs	Honey	Approx. relative value of sugar
1259-1400	28 lbs.	29 lbs.	34 doz.	—	150
1401-1540	20 lbs.	11 lbs.	19 doz.	12 lbs.	90
1541-1582	13 lbs.	7 lbs.	6 doz.	7 lbs.	45
1583-1702	3 lbs.	5 lbs.	4 doz.		20
1937	3 ozs.	3 ozs.	2 eggs	2½ ozs.	1

Source: *The History of Sugar,* Volume II, Noel Deerr.

in prices is shown in Table V. In 1902 an international agreement at Brussels prohibited countries represented from importing sugar on which a bounty was paid. The position was greatly eased, but not for long, and in 1928 the British Government adjusted the scale of sugar duties in such a way as to penalise the import of white sugar.

And so let us come up to the present day, with a look at the recent sugar trade of this country, which is shown in Tables VI and VII.

Table V: *Price of Raw Sugar in London, 1872-1904*

Year	Per Cwt.		Year	Per Cwt.		Year	Per Cwt.	
	s.	d.		s.	d.		s.	d.
1872	25	6	1883	19	0	1894	11	3
1873	22	6	1884	13	3	1895	10	0
1874	21	6	1885	11	9	1896	10	9
1875	20	0	1886	11	9	1897	9	3
1876	21	6	1887	11	9	1898	9	6
1877	24	6	1888	13	0	1899	10	6
1878	20	0	1889	16	0	1900	11	3
1879	19	0	1890	13	0	1901	9	3
1880	20	6	1891	13	0	1902	7	3
1881	21	3	1892	13	6	1903	8	6
1882	20	0	1893	14	0	1904	10	3

There are in Britain today three sugar producers and refiners — the British Sugar Corporation, with 26 per cent of the country's trade, the Manbre & Garton group, with 14 per cent, and Tate & Lyle, with 60 per cent. It may be of interest that of all the sugar consumed in the country, approximately one-half only is sold for domestic use over the grocer's counter and an equal quantity goes to the food manufacturing industries. The old pattern of packing sugar in bags and sacks is changing and an increasing number of industries call for their sugar in liquid form or have installed the plant to store and handle granulated sugar in bulk.

Table VI: *The Sugar Trade of Great Britain 1967*

Imported		Consumption		Refined Exports
Commonwealth Cane	1,793,000			
Foreign: Cane) Beet) White)	487,000			
	2,280,000		1,900,000	355,000
		Home Grown Beet	976,000	
			2,876,000	

ISC Metric Tons
     Raw Value 96° POL
     1967

Table VII: *Imported Sugars – UK Sources 1967*

000's Tons

1) Commonwealth
Australia	441		
Mauritius	376		
Caribbean	660		
Fiji	147		
India	78		
Swaziland	88	1,789	
Natal		161	1,950

2) Foreign
Cane:	Brazil	18		
	Cuba	81		
	Dominica	10		
	Other	114		
		223		
Beet:	E. Europe	37		
Refined		48		308
				2,258

6 THE LONDON MILK TRADE, 1900-1930

EDITH WHETHAM

In an earlier article,[1] I explored the organisation of the London market for liquid milk in the forty years between 1860 and 1900; here I propose to describe the changes which took place in the subsequent thirty years, until the Milk Marketing Boards were created under the Agricultural Marketing Acts of the 1930s. It may be useful first to summarise the main features of the London milk market as it existed in the railway age, before general use of motor transport.

In country districts, small towns and the suburbs of the cities, milk was sold to householders from hand carts or horse floats by retailers who were either producers of the milk sold, or direct buyers from the local farmers. Farmers might themselves deliver milk to the retailer's dairy, or they might drive their milk to the nearest railway station for consignment to the town station indicated by the buyer. The London market, serving a population of some six and a half millions, had already developed beyond this stage of direct contact between farmers and retailers still to be found in outer suburbs. The central area drew its supplies of milk from outside this ring, importing milk by railway fifty miles or more from Essex and Suffolk, from the south-eastern clover fields, from Wiltshire, east Dorset and Somerset, and from the Midlands as far north as Derbyshire, where the demands of London began to infringe on the milk sheds of the Lancashire towns. At railway stations in these dairying districts, wholesalers had built depots and creameries, where the milk was cooled before despatch by rail to London, and the seasonal surplus manufactured into various products. This manufacturing plant was subsidiary to the primary function of selling liquid milk to the London retailers and a response to the varying deliveries of the farmers.[2]

As the London wholesalers pushed westwards in search of supplies for their expanding market, they drew into the liquid trade farmers producing from summer grass milk which had customarily been converted into butter and cheese, either on the farms or in local factories. The production of winter milk required autumn-calving cows, fodder crops and purchased concentrates, all of which raised costs in comparison with the grass farms with their high output from April onwards and negligible sales in the winter months. Wholesalers also came into competition with the processors, who bought the cheap summer milk for manufacture; their factories were concentrated in Dorset, Devon, Somerset, west Wiltshire, Derbyshire and Staffordshire, in the areas where the London wholesale prices minus

65

the cost of rail transport to London ceased to provide a profitable market for the local dairy farmers.

The need for many farmers to dispose of their spring flush of milk, and the need of wholesalers to secure their supplies in the winter, had created by 1900 the six-monthly contract between the two parties. For the summer half-year, farmers' prices were relatively low, 5d. or 6d. a gallon, corresponding to the pressure to sell; in the winter half-year, prices might rise by 3d. or 4d. a gallon, corresponding to the pressure to buy. Farmers offering level deliveries over the season normally obtained rather higher prices than were offered by wholesalers for 'whole dairies' with varying outputs; producer-retailers, and retailers without manufacturing plant, required level supplies, but might also buy from, or sell to, the local wholesalers, as the occasion required. Railway stations, especially those in central London, had a brisk trade in milk churns, as local retailers adjusted their day's taking to the requirements of their customers.

The summer surplus over liquid consumption was often manufactured by the wholesalers at a financial loss, in spite of the low buying prices, since processing plant was seldom fully used. The wholesalers balanced their income over the year by selling to retailers at fairly level prices, irrespective of the season. Retailers equally charged their customers a level price, usually 4d. a quart in London and 3d. elsewhere, with appropriate discounts to institutional buyers and caterers who took milk in churns and not in quarts and pints. The customary high margin in the summer months encouraged competition from new traders, but they could not continue in business unless they also controlled adequate supplies for the winter trade and manufacturing plant to deal with the summer surplus which accompanied the winter sales. Moreover, the regular delivery of milk, once, twice daily, gave a decided advantage to the established retailers with compact blocks of customers; competition from new retailers commonly developed in the new suburbs rather than in the town centres. In the first decade of the new century, the London trade in liquid milk, of enormous importance to farmers south of the Trent, had thus settled into a stable pattern of semi-monopolistic competition, stable prices to the consumers subject to periodic price-cutting, and a recognised though varied pattern of prices paid by wholesalers to the farmers who supplied the basic raw material.

Milk consumption took other forms, however, than buying liquid milk from the roundsman. Condensed milk became increasingly popular in the last quarter of the nineteenth century, especially in the poorer families. Some was produced in Britain and there was a rising volume of imports. Sweetened condensed milk was both cheaper than fresh milk, if diluted to the same consistency, and it also kept longer, an important matter in houses with no larders. Condensed skimmed milk was cheaper still and was much used, it was feared, for feeding infants. But many families never tasted fresh milk; they took their milk already sweetened out of tins, thick or thin, according to the state of the family income.

Pure Milk and Public Opinion

With the increasing distance from which milk was drawn into central London came the twin problems of souring and the prevention of adulteration. Since householders could not rely on milk to keep overnight, the first delivery in the day might begin before 6 a.m., supplying milk direct from the railway station for breakfast. London firms advertised that they waited on families three times daily, thus inflicting a working day of 13 or 14 hours upon their roundsmen, reduced on Sundays by omitting the last delivery. Another method of coping with the problem of sour milk was to cool it. This became a function of the country depots, while some of the town dairies were installing cold rooms large enough to chill milk in churns. But in the hot summers of 1893 and 1911 towns were generally short of milk, partly because milk yields fell but mainly because milk could not be delivered before it went sour.

By 1910, a few firms had adopted either pasteurisation or sterilisation as a third method of reducing souring. Pasteurisation might be carried out at country depots, since it improved the quality of milk products as well as lengthening the life of milk destined for the liquid market. It might also be carried out in the town dairies, when milk might also be bottled for sale. Until the 1920s, however, pasteurised milk was commonly delivered in the usual manner, dipped from a churn into jugs provided by the buyers. Some firms supplied small cans with locking lids for their fussier consumers subject to periodic price-tarnished brass handles had been suspended in clusters on the railings', as described by Arnold Bennet in *Riceyman Steps,* published in 1923. Sterilising, favoured in the midland and northern towns, required the milk to be bottled and then boiled, with the bottles closed by glass tops and wire fasteners, adapted from the ginger-beer trade. Bottling further prevented adulteration of milk by roundsmen, one of the common plagues of the retailers who were liable to be summoned and fined for offences committed anywhere in the chain of distribution. But the supply of bottles, their collection, cleaning and capping, were expensive processes, only possible in the better-class trade where the distributive margin was protected by imperfect competition.

By 1910, some wholesalers and the larger retailers were also testing milk on purchase both for adulteration and for infection by bacteria; but churns despatched unsealed by train to London, sealed churns opened for testing, and churns taken out by roundsmen were continuously liable both to adulteration and to contamination. Nevertheless, regular testing at some stage in the distributive chain had its educational influence on both the original sellers of the milk and on the distributors. There was also the legal sanction of the Milk and Dairies Order, 1901, which established 3.0 per cent of butter-fat and 8.5 per cent of solids not fat as minima below which milk was presumed to be adulterated unless the seller could prove otherwise. It was an offence to sell milk judged unfit for human consumption.

In spite of these elementary precautions, there was increasing concern over the state of milk supplied in the years before and during the First World War. The trouble started with unhealthy cows, insanitary cowsheds, the lack of clean water and the lack of hygiene by the distributors. When hospitals began to test their milk, they were alarmed to find massive infection with 'B. Coli' and other impurities. In 1916-17, twenty out of thirty samples of milk delivered to Manchester hospitals carried more than one million bacteria per cc. Milk supplied through infant welfare centres in London to mothers and babies in the same year was also generally contaminated.[3]

The introduction of tuberculin tests in these years also revealed that varying proportions of the cows in the tested herds were infected with tuberculosis, and the infection was rampant in herds supplying winter milk. Of 750 samples of milk taken by inspectors at London railway stations in October-December 1913, 10 per cent were found to contain active tuberculosis.[4] These facts provoked a continuing argument about the connection between bovine and human forms of this disease. It was argued that they were not caused by the same organisms, and therefore could not be transmitted from one species to the other; alternatively, tuberculosis of the lungs was the most common form of infection in human beings, but drinking infected milk would, it was thought, lead to lesions in human stomachs, a comparatively rare disease.[5] Public opinion had however deduced a sufficient connection between both forms of tuberculosis for the government to have prohibited the sale of milk from cows with tuberculosis of the udder. Yet a London inspector visiting 64 farms supplying milk to his borough found seven such cows.[6]

One of the most striking features of any spell of hot weather in the nineteenth century was the rise in infant mortality ascribed to 'summer diarrhoea'. There was a particularly bad epidemic in the hot years of the later 1890s, followed by a marked peak in the drought of 1911. In London the infant mortality from all causes in the third quarter of the year rose from 91 per 1,000 births in 1910 to 203 in 1911, and fell back to 83 in the cool summer of 1912.[7] Infected milk was one obvious factor here, and the gradual improvement in milk hygiene during the twentieth century undoubtedly contributed to the marked fall in the infant death rate.

The enforcement of regulations about the hygiene of milk

was hindered, in the years before the First World War, partly by the ignorance of farmers and dairymen, partly by the apathy of most of the public, but also by the multiplicity of authorities, each dealing with a limited area. Inspectors of London boroughs had authority only over the milk sold within their borough's boundaries. Wholesalers and retailers with depots and shops scattered over London were expected to register in every borough, but often omitted this formality. When summoned for selling adulterated or unfit milk, it was difficult for the sellers to trace the offending consignment through the distributive chain to the distant area whence it originated, where the farms would in any event come under a sanitary board dominated by the farmer members of county councils. Many city and county boroughs tried to obtain special powers under private bills to exercise authority over farms supplying milk sold within their boundaries. They were consistently opposed by the Chambers of Agriculture and later by the newly-formed National Farmers' Unions, who argued that legislation over milk must be uniformly applied over all the country and not left to the overlapping powers of local authorities.

Measures to improve the quality and hygiene of the milk supply were initiated mainly by the wholesalers and the larger retailers who were concerned with prolonging the life, and promoting the sales, of a perishable article. It was these firms which pushed ahead with the regular testing of milk, with the education of their supplying farmers, and with the installation of pasteurising and bottling plant, sometimes doing so with the encouragement of the local medical officers of health. Farmers and the smaller distributors were generally apathetic or opposed to such innovations, partly because of the fear of rising costs and partly because of the dislike of increasing interference by inspectors of all types. Moreover, the medical profession was itself divided upon the value of pasteurising or sterilising milk. The Committee which investigated the physical condition of the nation after the Boer War found that some doctors rejected sterilised milk as lacking in nutritive qualities. There was evidence that infants fed entirely upon it developed scurvy and rickets, and also that calves so fed did not thrive normally.[8] In addition, pasteurisation was often imperfectly carried out and milk could then be reinfected by the process. Pure milk from healthy cows, properly cooled before transport, bottled and promptly delivered, was the objective of many reformers, and pasteurisation could well obscure this progress.

Costs, Combines and Nationalisation

Whatever the conflicts of medical opinion, experience showed the necessity for pasteurisation, as the London wholesalers reached further into Dorset, Somerset, Devon and South Wales in order to gather enough milk for the expanding London market which was threatened by periodic shortages in the winter months. By 1914, the London trade was dominated by four or five wholesalers, equipped with country depots, a huge supply of churns, regular contracts with the railways, pasteurising plant and cold stores in their town dairies. These firms were the Wiltshire United Dairies, under their London manager, Joseph Maggs; the Great Western and Metropolitan Dairies, a combination of firms controlled by the Butler and Price families; the Dairy Supply Company, the wholesaling subsidiary of the Express Dairies, managed by the Barham dynasty; and F.W. Gilbert, which had originated in Derbyshire. The Eastern Counties Dairy Farmers' Society, one of the few farmers' co-operatives in the London market, and the consumer co-operatives, stood rather outside the wholesale market for milk, though they competed with the wholesalers for farm contracts, and with retailers for their customers. The co-operative societies had little manufacturing plant and thus required level deliveries from their suppliers.

Within a few months of the outbreak of war, there were shortages of roundsmen in London, and a shortage of feeding stuffs for the cows; the supply of milk began to fall and with rising wages added to rising costs of purchases, milk prices to the consumers rose sharply in 1915 and 1916. Maximum retail prices were imposed in November 1916, limiting increases to stated proportions above those which had been charged in the corresponding months in the pre-war years, thus preserving the diversity of actual prices between towns and country and between retailers offering different qualities of milk or different types of service.

In the summer of 1915, the managers of the Wiltshire United Dairies combined with the Price, Barham and Gilbert families to create United Dairies, controlling at the time of its formation possibly half the wholesale trade in milk in London. The proclaimed object of the combine was to maintain distribution by the rationalising of deliveries of milk from wholesalers to the retailers' premises with economies in horses and men. Within eighteen months, the new firm had raised a capital of £1 million, and its managing director, R.R.F. Butler, emphasised the numbers of premises closed, men and horses released for other work, and the costs eliminated, at a time when the general rise in prices was causing hardship among the poorer families.

The dominating influence of the combine aroused alarm among the London retailers, which intensified with rumours in 1917 that the firm was buying up retailers as well as other wholesalers. In May 1918, under pressure from the Ministry of Food, United Dairies published a list of nearly one hundred firms, wholesale and retail, which it had either bought or was in the process of buying.[9] Here again the objective was stated to be economies in horses, dairies, equipment and roundsmen which alone could enable distribution to be maintained under the controlled margins.

The 'milk combine' was at once attacked in the House of Commons as a dangerous monopoly, alleged to control at the end of the war some two-thirds of the wholesale trade in London, and about one-third of the retail trade.[10] The Astor Committee, appointed in April 1917 to enquire into the production and distribution of milk, was impressed both by the further economies which could follow a still more drastic rationalisation of milk transport, and by the power of the combine over the supply of milk to London and the southern half of England. The Committee recommended[11] that the Government should take immediate control of the supply of milk, as it had of the supply of other foods, appointing the existing firms as its agents with controlled margins. Further, it suggested that the Government should acquire options to buy out the existing firms after the war, thus nationalising the distribution of milk and ensuring that the benefits of rationalisation would accrue to consumers in the form of lower prices, and not to the owners of the combine in the form of larger profits. Such municipalities as wished might also be allowed to organise the retail distribution of milk within their boundaries as a public service. In May 1918, the Government accepted the recommendations of the Astor Committee, and issued two Orders authorising the Ministry of Food to take over, from a date to be determined, the premises and plant engaged in milk distribution. The chief architect of the combine, Butler of the United Dairies, was brought on to the new Milk Control Board to show the Government how to run this new nationalised industry.[12]

The project, however, aroused intense opposition, from farmers who feared a single national wholesaler even more than the existing firms; from retailers and producer-retailers, uncertain of their ability to buy and sell marginal quantities, even if they survived 'municipalisation'; and from manufacturers of milk products, who saw the national wholesaler as an all-powerful competitor in the markets in which they bought their raw material and in the markets in which they sold their output. Moreover, the efforts of the Ministry of Food to find a rational basis for fixing prices to farmers had foundered on the absence of reliable costings for the production of milk. 'The opinions of the agricultural experts were so divergent that it is impossible to treat them in the light of reliable evidence. The Ministry in fixing prices, had before them estimates ranging from $2s.9d.$ to $4s.9d.$ per gallon.'[13] It was possible for a year or two to fix maximum prices in relation to ascertained changes in certain costs such as cattle cake and wages, but this would hardly be adequate as a payment policy of a nationalised wholesaler, responsible to Parliament, to consumers of liquid milk and to the farmers themselves.

These problems only rose above the horizon to sink again from view. After a winter of argument, nationalisation of the milk trade was swept into oblivion by the Armistice, and the change in government which followed; the project was officially abandoned in a statement to the Commons on 2 July 1919. The Milk Control Board died at the same time, having dealt with the shortage of milk in the winter of 1918-19 by the rationing of wholesalers and retailers, and by the fixing of higher prices on purchase from farmers. The milk combine was, however, referred to the Standing Committee on Trusts, under the Profiteering Acts, 1919 and 1920, whose report stated the problem which was to be argued over in the years between the wars.[14] United Dairies and the remaining large wholesalers such as Express Dairies undoubtedly had lower costs than the smaller firms, whether in wholesaling or in retailing. They therefore could make handsome profits from the prices required to keep their competitors in existence. A fall in the distributive margin would cheapen milk to the consumers, by driving out of business the producer-retailers and numerous small retailers, leaving half a dozen firms and the consumer co-operatives in control of the London milk market.

Public Health and the Promotion of Consumption

By 1925, 'practically the whole of the milk sold in London was pasteurised',[15] either by the wholesalers or the consumer cooperatives. The medical objection to heat-treated milk disappeared with the further knowledge of vitamins and of the value of orange juice and cod liver oil in supplying what might be lacking in milk. Nevertheless, compulsory pasteurisation was still opposed for two main reasons. Firstly, it would eliminate from the retail market the producer-retailers and many small retailers buying direct from farmers, thus strengthening the position of the large firms who alone could afford to install the necessary plant. Although necessary for the London trade, pasteurisation and bottling would probably raise costs and prices in the country districts. Secondly, Stenhouse Williams and others at the University of Reading and elsewhere argued that compulsory pasteurisation would deter farmers from producing clean milk from healthy cows guaranteed free of tuberculosis and that distributors would be unwilling to pay the higher prices prescribed since 1922 for clean milk from certified herds if all milk was bulked for pasteurisation before sale.[16] All through the inter-war years, the pasteurisers and the campaigners for clean milk argued against each other, but they did at least educate farmers and the consumer public in the value of clean milk reasonably free from harmful bacteria.

The progress of improvement in milk supplied is difficult to trace outside the main towns, since each area had its own history, depending on the enthusiasm of the medical officers of health and the enterprise of local retailers and farmers. Students of local history may be interested to find out when milk in their district was first sold in bottles and by whom; which firm installed the first plant for pasteurising or sterilising milk; which producer-retailers won prizes for clean milk or were the earliest to have herds certified free of tuberculosis; and when the independent retailers gave up buying their own milk and bought from a pasteurising wholesaler.

Making milk safe to drink, by whatever method, was particularly important when it came to promoting its consumption. Much evidence had been given to the 1904 Inter-Departmental Committee on Physical Deterioration on the inadequate feeding of many children in the elementary schools.[17] One result was the institution of school meals and of welfare centres for providing cheap milk to mothers and children under school age. In 1918, when the retail prices of milk in London rose to 10*d.* a quart, more than double the pre-war prices, local authorities were allowed to provide milk free or at reduced prices to the priority consumers, but only a few towns inflicted such a cost upon their rates. The association of poverty and low consumption of milk was brought out by many social studies between the wars. Notable among these was the investigation published in 1936 by Boyd Orr, *Food, Health and Income,* in which the late E.M.H. Lloyd played an important part. Milk consumption varied not only with income but also with dietary customs; generally speaking, only children and invalids drank milk by itself during these years, while adults consumed milk mainly in hot drinks and cooked foods.

The Milk Market After the First World War

Statistics on the production of milk and dairy products in Great Britain derive from the census of production taken in 1907-8, 1924-5 and 1930-31. Of the amount of milk sold liquid from farms at the first census, it was thought that possibly one-quarter or more was manufactured by the buyers. (see Table I).

The period of milk control also produced some imperfect statistics which suggested that sales off farms fell from about 1,253 million gallons in 1914 to less than a thousand million gallons in 1919, as a result of the ploughing up of grassland and the shortage of cattle feeds. Apart from these war years, it appears that the consumption of liquid milk per head showed little change during the first thirty years of the century, but this stationary average concealed wide variations in consumption between areas and income groups; the wartime control indicated that some northern towns had an average consumption of about one-tenth of a pint per head per day, compared with one-third of a pint in the wealthiest districts of the south-east.[18]

Table I: *Use of Milk Sold in Great Britain*

Million gallons milk	1907-8	1924-5	1930-31
Estimated sales off farms	1,064	1,035	1,158
Sold liquid	850	788	874
as butter	140	164	186
as cheese	56	73	77
as cream	18	10	21
Of amount sold liquid			
made into butter	–	14	25
cheese	–	24	60
cream	–	31	25
condensed & dried	–	37	42
waste	–	38	43
consumed as liquid	–	644	679

Agricultural Output 1907-8, Cd. 6277, 1912; Report, Reorganisation Commission for Milk, Min. Agric. Econ. Series 38, 1933.

From 1920 onwards, prices fell sharply in all sectors of the market, and more slowly from 1922 onwards. In the mid-1920s, farmers selling milk to London wholesalers were receiving prices 60-70 per cent above those ruling in 1914, while the London retail prices settled down at much the same relative level, at about 6*d.* or 6½*d.* a quart, compared with 4*d.* before the war.[19] There were however continuing changes in the organisation of the market.

In the first place, the various parties to the milk trade had necessarily created representative bodies to negotiate with governments, firstly, over the Milk and Dairies Orders, and secondly, over the wartime controls. Just before the war, the London wholesalers had formed the National Federation of Dairymens' Associations, which brought closer contacts with those larger retailers from the midland towns who were also buyers from farmers. This association was dominated after 1915 by United Dairies. The smaller firms in London revived the Metropolitan Dairymen's Association and also formed the Amalgamated Master Dairymen, partly to resist the extension of the combine. Retailers outside London were also represented in discussions with the Government by the Chambers of Agriculture and later by the National Farmers' Unions.

In the disorganised market of 1921, a joint Committee of the NFU and the NFDA attempted to work out agreed prices for the London trade. Thereafter, this Permanent Joint Committee negotiated standard six-monthly contracts with recommended prices which were widely publicised. Although each farmer and buyer continued to make their own terms, at least the parties had a guide to current ideas of market prices. There remained however a wide variation in the actual prices received by farmers, as was shown by a study of 80 milk-selling farms in the Blackmore Vale.[20] For the winter of 1928-9, prices received, after deduction of transport charges, ranged from 15½d. per gallon to 11½d.; in the following summer, the variation ran from 13d. down to 7½d. This surprising variation, even in one small area, was caused partly by differences in transport charges, partly by differences in the seasonality and quality of output, and partly by the bargaining ability of the farmers. Adjacent farmers selling milk to the same buyer and paying the same haulier seldom cooperated over their bargaining, partly for fear of revealing to each other the size of their incomes. Prewett noticed that the farmers supplying the five retailers in Glastonbury sold separately through one wholesaler.[21] Transport charges were especially variable as motor lorries began to operate either from independent hauliers or as part of the buyers' services, paid for by a deduction from the monthly milk cheque. The short journeys from farm to retailer or to the country depot were increasingly transferred to road haulage, leaving only the long-distance trade to continue from country railway stations to the London terminals, and even this was eroded in the 1930s by the development of road tankers. Moreover, road transport brought into the milk market many farms previously out of reach of any railway station.

The mid-1920s saw the end of the tripartite structure which had begun to evolve in the London market in the 1860s, with competing wholesalers buying from farmers and selling to retailers. The reasons for the amalgamation of wholesaling and retailing lie in the changing technology of the trade, in the introduction of pasteurisation, refrigeration and the bottling plant. These processes required expensive equipment, the bulking of supplies to obtain economies of scale, and the minimum of transport in the chain from collecting depot to the final buyers. The dominating influence of railway transport and of the markets in accommodating milk at the London stations faded away, as a few large firms organised the flow of a perishable and vulnerable commodity through their sub-departments. Prices and profit margins came increasingly under the influence of collective bargaining, with the United Dairies and Express Dairies as the dominant buyers for the London trade throughout southern England, the western counties, into Cornwall and Carmarthenshire, and up into the midland valleys. There was still competition from the consumer cooperative societies, from the large number of producer-retailers and small retailers, and from the independent manufacturers of milk products, but these all tended to follow, rather than to upset, the prices set by the large firms. This pattern of small and large firms linked by imperfect competition was broken by the onset of the great depression in 1929-30, with the subsequent collapse of milk prices and the hurried birth of the Milk Marketing Boards as monopoly wholesalers operating on behalf of the milk-selling farmers.

Notes

1. E.H. Whetham, 'The London Milk Trade 1860-1900', *Econ. Hist. Rev.*, 2nd ser. XVII (1964), pp.369-80.
2. See the map of creameries given in R.B. Forrester, 'Fluid Milk Market in England and Wales', Min. of Agric. Econ. series 16, HMSO, 1927.
3. Astor Committee on the Production and Distribution of Milk, Final Report, pp.12, 77, Cd. 9095, 1918.
4. *Cowkeeper and Dairyman's Journal,* Feb. 1914, p.258.
5. F.J. Lloyd, 'How can Tuberculosis Best be Eliminated from Dairy Herds of a Country', *Journal British Dairy Farmers' Assoc.,* 1908, pp.75-7; N. Raw, 'Human and Bovine Tuberculosis', *Brit. Med. J.,* 14 Mar. 1903, p.596.
6. *Cowkeeper and Dairyman's Journal,* Feb. 1914, p.258.
7. 'Report on Infant and Child Mortality', Local Government Board, Cd. 5263, 1910 and Cd. 6909, 1913.
8. 'Report of the Inter-Departmental Committee on Physical Deterioration', pp.54, 55, 449, HMSO, 1904.
9. *Cowkeeper and Dairyman's Journal,* Aug. 1917, p.463; May 1918, p.215.
10. Hansard, 1918, March 29; May 13; June 26; July 3.
11. Astor Committee on the Production and Distribution of Milk, Final Report, Cd. 9095, 1918.
12. W.H. Beveridge, *British Food Control,* London, 1928, p.271.
13. Beveridge, op. cit., p.171, quoting the report of a committee of investigation set up by the Food Control Committees in 1919.
14. 'Report on Milk by the Standing Committee on Trusts', Cd. 1102, 1920.
15. F.J. Prewett, *Marketing of Farm Produce,* II, Milk, Oxford, 1927, p.23.
16. Forrester, loc. cit., p.46.
17. 'Report of the Inter-Departmental Committee on Physical Deterioration', HMSO, 1904.
18. See the tables on pp.15-16; also the 'Report of the Reorganisation Commission for Milk', pp.33-42, Min. of Agric. Econ. series 38, HMSO, 1933.
19. R.L. Cohen, *History of Milk Prices,* Oxford, 1936, gives the general story of these years.
20. G.B. Bisset, C. Pringle and E. Thomas, *Dairy Farming in the Blackmore Vale,* Dept. of Agric. Econ., Univ. of Reading, Survey Studies No. 1, Reading, 1931.
21. F.J. Prewett, *A Survey of Milk Marketing... in Wiltshire, Somerset, and the City of Bristol,* Oxford, 1928, p.36.

7 THE COCOA AND CHOCOLATE INDUSTRY IN THE NINETEENTH CENTURY

J. OTHICK

It is the purpose of this essay to outline the history of the cocoa and chocolate industry in Britain before 1914, and to indicate those factors which seem to have been most influential in the growth of the industry. At the same time, we hope to relate the experience of this industry to some of the more general themes and controversies associated with late nineteenth-century economic history. Our major area of concern will be the later nineteenth century, mainly because it is then that the cocoa and chocolate industry experienced its most significant growth and emerged for the first time as a large-scale manufacturing business. It will also be necessary to consider the industry in an international perspective, because foreign influences have played a decisive role in its development.

The cocoa bean, which originates in Latin America, was introduced into Europe by the Spanish in the sixteenth century. By the mid-seventeenth century, its use had spread to most of western Europe, including Britain. Perhaps the most convenient method of periodising the subsequent history of the British cocoa and chocolate industry is on the basis of the type of social market for which it catered. This method is necessarily arbitrary, and is intended merely as a general guide. During the first phase, from its introduction until the late eighteenth century, cocoa remained an expensive luxury item, available only to the rich. In the ensuing phase — which covers the first three-quarters of the nineteenth century — cocoa products were increasingly being consumed by the middle classes. And it is only during the third phase — from the last quarter of the nineteenth century onwards — that cocoa products have become articles of mass consumption. It is essential to understand that these phases in the evolution of the industry closely reflect changes in the nature of the product, which are in turn associated with changing technology.[1]

We can gain some general impression of the progress of the industry by considering the pattern of raw cocoa imports. It will be clear from Table I that there was a rapid and, for the most part, sustained increase in both gross and net imports of raw cocoa over the period of the later nineteenth century. It is necessary, of course, to relate these figures to the growth of population over the period, and to compare the experience of cocoa with that of other beverages. Table II indicates clearly that *per capita* consumption of cocoa products increased at a sharp pace throughout the period, although there was a perceptible decline in the growth rate after 1900. It can also be seen how consumption of cocoa products compared with the consumption of

Table I: *Annual Imports of Raw Cocoa into United Kingdom* (m. lbs.)

	Gross imports	Net imports
1870	14.8	6.9
1880	23.5	10.6
1890	28.1	20.2
1900	52.6	37.8
1910	70.1	53.1

Source: *Statistical Abstract for the United Kingdom.*

Table II: *Annual* per capita *Consumption of Tea, Coffee, and Cocoa* (lbs.)

	Tea	Coffee	Cocoa
1870	3.76	0.97	0.20
1880	4.57	0.92	0.30
1890	5.17	0.75	0.54
1900	6.07	0.71	0.92
1910	6.39	0.65	1.18

Source: B.R. Mitchell and P.M. Deane (eds.), *Abstract of British Historical Statistics,* 1962, pp.8-10.

other beverages. Tea was clearly a firmly established leader before 1870, whilst, on the other hand, coffee appears to have been declining in popularity.

It is normal to view the period of the late nineteenth century — at least until the mid-1890s — as a period of falling prices for primary commodities; and to see the increasing *per capita* consumption of various foodstuffs as a natural consequence of this trend. However, the increasing consumption of cocoa products cannot be explained in these terms. An index of wholesale prices is shown in Table III.

Table III: *Index of Wholesale Prices* (1900 = 100)

	Tea	Coffee	Cocoa
1870	192	94	72
1880	158	132	116
1890	125	138	100
1900	100	100	100
1910	93	83	102

Source: A.R. Prest and A.A. Adams, *Consumers' Expenditure in the United Kingdom, 1900-1919,* 1954.

It is clear that consumption of cocoa products increased at a time when there was no marked decline in prices; in fact, average prices were rising during the earlier part of the period, whilst remaining fairly static during the later part. This stands out in marked contrast to the experience of tea, where falling prices were obviously a significant factor contributing to the increase in consumption.

Apart from changes in its overall size, there were also changes in the structure and organisation of the cocoa and chocolate industry. In simple terms, production came increasingly to be concentrated in a small number of large firms; in fact, by the early twentieth century the industry was very much dominated by the three firms of Cadbury, Fry and Rowntree.[2] But this was the situation during the third phase in the industry's evolution — the period when it was beginning to penetrate working-class markets. It is necessary to ask how the transition from second to third phase occurred, to examine the factors that lie behind the growth of the industry up to and including the late nineteenth century.

The general thesis adduced here is that two factors, above all, have conditioned the development of the cocoa and chocolate industry: on the supply side, there was the nature and timing of technological innovation; and, on the demand side, there were the limitations imposed by restricted markets. The latter point is fairly easily explained. Whilst there existed a general deficiency of effective demand at the working-class level, the possibilities implicit in technological innovations could never be exploited fully: in this industry, we have an example — probably not an isolated one — where mass production was a possibility before a mass market had grown up.

When we come to analyse the supply side, we encounter an extremely complex situation. The first reason for this is that we are here dealing with an industry which was technologically precocious. From an early stage, cocoa processing had a much higher technical optimum than that for other industries involved in the processing of foodstuffs. In particular, this is true if we compare cocoa with the other non-alcoholic beverages — tea and coffee — both of which have continued to be processed in fairly small economic units right into the twentieth century. By comparison, cocoa processing was occurring on a factory basis from the early nineteenth century and even before. Even in the late eighteenth century, simple machines for crushing and milling were developed, and gradually the advantages of the small factory over the traditional workshop/retailing unit became apparent to the more energetic and ambitious entrepreneur. Fry's — the earliest of the large British firms to appear — installed a Boulton and Watt steam engine in their Bristol premises as early as 1795. The early decades of the nineteenth century saw the establishment on a factory basis of many of the firms which still dominate the European cocoa and chocolate industry: Menier in France in 1824; Suchard in Switzerland in 1826; Van Houten in Holland in 1828; and Cadbury in 1831. There even existed — from the late 1830s — engineering firms such as Lehmann of Dresden, which specialised in the manufacture of cocoa- and chocolate-processing machinery.

In spite of what has been said about the comparatively early date at which cocoa was manufactured on a factory basis, this should not obscure the fact that the diffusion of new techniques was slow, and that the typical business unit remained a small-scale affair throughout the first half of the nineteenth century. During these years, the functions of dealer, processor, and retailer were usually combined, whilst it was common for the business to have interests in tea and coffee as well as in cocoa. Even in the second half of the nineteenth century, the situation did not change rapidly, and the small workshop-type firm survived into the twentieth century, although the industry was by then dominated by a handful of large firms.

A second factor which has to be taken into consideration when we look at the supply side is that technological innovation brought about at an early stage a situation where two products — cocoa and chocolate — were obtained under fairly rigid conditions of joint supply. Apart from any problems associated with this joint supply situation, it was to have significant repercussions on the pattern of trade that developed — both within Europe, and between Europe and the raw material supplying countries.

A third point that has to be noted about the role of technology in this industry is that technical changes tended not so much to lower costs, but to make available better-quality products, or new types of product. This fact has to be seen in conjunction with a fourth point — and that is the slowness of diffusion of technology. Largely because of market limitations, new techniques diffused only slowly, thus giving rise to a series of short-term situations where one firm — or a small group of firms in one country — held a monopoly or near-monopoly position in the supply of one type of product — the one, that is, made possible by the particular technique pioneered by the firm in question. Again, this characteristic of technology was to have a marked influence on the trading pattern that emerged. Another point is that the slow diffusion of new techniques meant not only the survival of old techniques, but also the survival of old types of product. So — at any one time, and generally more so later in the century — there was subsumed under the title of cocoa a variety of different products, using different ingredients, produced by different methods, and catering for different markets. However, paradoxically, they were not necessarily produced by different firms: because it became possible to produce a new type of product, firms did not necessarily abandon lines which they already manufactured.

We have so far considered the nature and implications of technological change only in very general terms. It is worth looking more closely at some of the actual innovations that occurred in cocoa and chocolate technology. During the course of the nineteenth century, there were three major developments, each of them originating outside the United Kingdom — another point which has implications for the pattern of trade that was to emerge. The first was the process perfected by the Dutch firm of Van Houten in 1828, which made it possible to remove some of the fat content — usually referred to as cocoa-butter — from the cocoa bean. Before this, the normal practice had been to add some form of starch in order to counteract the fat. With the Van Houten process, it became possible on the one hand to produce an absolutely pure cocoa powder for drinking purposes; and, on the other hand, the cocoa-butter which had been removed could be used as a basis for manufacturing chocolate in a solid form. The important point is that the two products were unavoidably produced together in more or less fixed proportions; the only way in which the proportions could be varied was by using a grade, or a different species of cocoa bean, which would have a lower fat content.

Diffusion of the Van Houten process was slow, and it is clear that it was not widely used in England until the last third of the nineteenth century. This can be seen from the persistence of the old, adulterated[3] form of cocoa, even into the twentieth century. The nature of this type of product is indicated in contemporary advertisements, recipes, and patents: typically, the fat content of the cocoa bean was counteracted by adding, in varying proportions, items such as powdered lentils, tapioca, sago, or arrowroot. Contemporary descriptions would suggest that this type of cocoa had a closer resemblance to soup than to the sort of beverage we normally think of. 'A wholesome gruel' was a description applied to it by one of the Cadbury family.[4] It was produced mostly, and to a later date, by a proliferation of small firms operating in local markets, and employing obsolete techniques. However, even large, reputable firms like Rowntree and Cadbury, who had adopted the Van Houten technique in the 1860s, continued also to produce the adulterated type of cocoa until as late as 1890.

The fact that reputable firms continued to produce old, adulterated cocoa as well as the cocoa essence made possible by the new technique provides one important explanation for the slow spread of the new process: in simple terms, the old type of cocoa had come to enjoy a certain degree of popularity, and, to many palates, it was more acceptable than the new, pure cocoa. Another point that might be connected with this is that many people drank cocoa not so much because they liked it, but because they thought it possessed certain medicinal properties. In other words, if they believed the old cocoa to be having the desired effect, then they probably saw no reason to change their brand.[5] There were, of course, other explanations for the slow spread of the Van Houten process. For one thing, Van Houten had every reason to keep the technique to themselves. Another point is that, partly because of the joint supply problem the pure cocoa was more expensive than the adulterated cocoa. In short, manufacturers could not hope to exploit wider markets — that is, lower-income groups — until there was some substantial improvement in the standard of living of the mass of the people — arguably, something which occurred on a sufficient scale only from the 1870s onwards. Similarly, of course, the producer of the cheapest and poorest-quality cocoa could survive as long as there were social groups which could not afford anything better. Finally, we cannot afford to overlook the ignorance and conservatism of many entrepreneurs as a possible explanation for the slow spread of the Van Houten method.

The second innovation that affected profoundly the development of the industry concerned the manufacture of cocoa powder, and may be seen as a refinement to the original Van Houten process. Again, the Dutch were the pioneers, and the process — which dates from the 1860s — involved adding alkali during the processing of the cocoa in order to make the cocoa powder more easily soluble. The important thing is that small amounts of the alkali remained in the finished product, and affected its taste. For reasons which are difficult to discern, the new type of cocoa proved more acceptable to most palates, and the old product was gradually supplanted. The success of the alkaline variety of cocoa probably owed much to the fact that it was pioneered by Van Houten, who were already a well-established name in a wide range of markets. The major British firms were at first reluctant to use the new method because they maintained that it represented a return to adulteration, and that the absolutely pure cocoa essence could not be improved upon. However, they were eventually forced to follow suit when it became clear that the alkaline cocoa was proving more popular than the pure cocoa.

The late nineteenth century presents a complicated picture as regards the manufacture of cocoa. Because of the slowness of diffusion, there were three distinct types of product, drunk largely by different income groups, each representing a different phase in the technological evolution of the industry: there was the old, adulterated cocoa produced by pre-Van Houten methods; there was the pure cocoa — or cocoa essence — which had been made possible by the Van Houten process; and there was the new, alkaline cocoa. Long before the second type had supplanted the first, it was itself being supplanted by the third.

The third of the major technological developments of the nineteenth century concerned the manufacture of milk chocolate. In this case, the Swiss[6] were the pioneers, and it was in the 1870s that the first milk chocolate appeared. Again, diffusion was slow — probably for much the same reasons as in the case of the Van Houten process — and it was not until the turn of the century that British manufacturers first successfully produced milk chocolate, although they had strenuously been trying to do so for many years. However, it is possible to argue that, even if the technique had spread to Britain sooner, manufacturers would still have faced a market situation where demand was effectively confined to the better-off social classes. The experience of Cadbury's would seem to lend some support to this point of view. The first line in moulded chocolate to enjoy major and lasting success was their Dairy Milk brand, which was a best-seller in the years before 1914. By contrast, earlier lines marketed by this firm do not seem to have met with much success in finding a mass market. On the other hand, there is evidence from the firm of Fry's that various lines in moulded chocolate had been successful in penetrating mass markets well before the turn of the century.

The growth of the cocoa and chocolate industry in the nineteenth century was accompanied by the development of a particularly complex pattern of international trade. This was something which was at least partly a result of technological changes; it also stemmed from the lack of a mass market for cocoa products during much of the century. At two levels, technology and the pattern of demand affected international trading patterns: at one level, it is necessary to consider intra-European trading patterns; at another level, it is necessary to consider the changing relationship between the major manufacturing countries and their suppliers of raw materials.

There are several reasons why cocoa products came from an early stage to feature in trade between various European countries. For one thing, they remained luxury products for much of the nineteenth century, and luxury products tend naturally to have wider geographical markets. Another reason for the growth of trade is simply that the major innovations occurred in small countries with only limited local markets: it was only natural that the Dutch and the Swiss should try to exploit the larger and richer markets of the major industrial nations. A third point is that, because of slow diffusion, the pioneer firm could continue to exploit its advantage in foreign markets for a long time after the original innovation, thus building up a momentum in its foreign trade. This certainly happened with Van Houten and with the Swiss manufacturers of milk chocolate. Probably until as late as the 1890s, Van Houten sold more cocoa in Britain than any single British firm. As early as the 1870s, Van Houten had agencies in London, Leeds, Liverpool, Edinburgh, Glasgow, and Dublin — at a time, that is, when firms like Rowntree and Cadbury were only just beginning to move towards establishing a nation-wide distributive network. When we look at the example of milk chocolate, we again find an enormous level of imports into Britain, particularly after the turn of the century.[7] A fourth reason for the growth of intra-European trade relates to consumer preferences: it would seem that, where luxury goods are concerned, consumers tend to be more irrational. Swiss chocolate continued to be exported to Britain for long after British substitutes of similar quality and price had become available, which seems to indicate that the Swiss, once having gained a strong hold on this type of trade, could not easily be challenged. Whilst manufacturers had to rely on a stratum of society where quality — real or imagined — was far more important than cost, there seems to have been a tendency for the innovator to gain a more or less unassailable position. This could not be eroded until lower-cost producers could tap new markets at lower social levels — which is precisely what Cadbury's achieved with their Dairy Milk line in the years before 1914.

A final reason for the growth of intra-European trade in cocoa products is the joint supply problem. This meant that, unless identical local market situations obtained for both cocoa and chocolate, the producer was faced with the need to find foreign outlets for whichever was least in demand locally. It so happened that Van Houten found themselves able to sell much larger quantities of cocoa than of chocolate — which remained a more expensive luxury item for much longer. Consequently, throughout the middle decades of the nineteenth century, the Dutch were releasing large quantities of cocoa-butter on to European markets, much of it finding its way to French chocolate manufacturers. This assisted a process of international specialisation in which the French soon emerged as the leading producers of high-quality chocolate assortments. One firm in particular stood out in this type of trade, and that was the firm of Menier. This firm's output rose from in the region of 500,000 kilograms per annum in the 1850s to 10 million kilograms per annum by the 1870s.[8] For the various reasons which have already been considered, this was a heavily export-oriented trade, with Britain becoming one of the most important foreign markets. In fact, Menier found it worth while to open a subsidiary factory in London in 1870, such was the size of their British business. One lasting result of this development was the French emphasis in the luxury chocolate trade in Britain. This is why French names like crème, praline, or nougat are still so commonly used in chocolate assortments. Cadbury's for many years found it desirable to have a Paris address; and it has even been suggested that the name 'Bourneville' reflects the French influence.

The main point we are making is that the foreign influence — whether French, Dutch or Swiss — has been important, and is only a reflection of a complex trading pattern, where large quantities of cocoa products at varying stages of manufacture were crossing European frontiers. In the early years, this was more a flow into Britain than out of it;[9] but, at a much later date, overseas connections began to offer opportunities which the more successful British firms could exploit.

The outward-looking nature of the industry is seen in the fact that there was an international conference of cocoa and chocolate manufacturers as early as 1911 — a much earlier date than in most other industries.

The other level at which changing patterns of international trade need to be considered is in terms of the relationship between manufacturing countries and raw material suppliers. Initially, Latin America was the only source of cocoa beans, but, during the middle decades of the nineteenth century, increasing quantities began to come from the Portuguese islands of Sao Thome and Principe off the coast of West Africa, in the Gulf of Guinea. Probably fortuitously, the type of cocoa bean that was cultivated in these islands was of a poor grade, with a low fat content. Because of the joint supply situation, and because cocoa was more in demand in Europe than chocolate, there was a preference on the part of many manufacturers for low grade fruit. This resulted in an enormous growth of imports from Portuguese West Africa, and, ultimately, from the mainland of Africa itself. In short, technology and the nature of markets within Europe eventually brought about a complete change in the major source of raw materials, with West Africa eventually taking over from Latin America.[10]

We have so far concentrated very much on the supply side, and we hope to have shown that technological bottlenecks were not a problem: the problem was more one of finding markets for the products that technology made available. It was precisely because of this problem that the complex international trading situation developed; and it was because of this problem that we find the coexistence of different types of product using different techniques. By the time we reach the late nineteenth century, the problem is clearly in the process of being solved. And — when we come to ask why — the answer must surely be found on the demand side.

At the simplest level of analysis, we have to look at the changing demand situation for cocoa products in terms of an income effect and a substitution effect. People were buying more cocoa products either because they were better-off, or because they were spending less money on other products. The most obvious answer is that real wages were increasing because of falling prices: cocoa was simply another item in a list of consumer goods that the mass of the population could for the first time afford — a list which includes items such as sugar, soap, tobacco, and perhaps bicycles, sewing-machines or pianos. Yet this is not the whole answer, otherwise it would be possible to show a much closer correlation between levels of real wages and consumption of cocoa products. The rate of increase of *per capita* consumption does slow down after the turn of the century,[11] which is when we would expect it to if we are relating cocoa consumption to real wages. However, this slowing down is a long way from the stagnation in real wages that has been observed during the Edwardian period. We are therefore persuaded that there must also have been some kind of substitution effect.

Of the various reasons for believing this, perhaps the most persuasive is the growth of temperance, and the declining *per capita* consumption of alcohol. There is no doubt that there did occur a downturn in *per capita* consumption of drink towards the end of the nineteenth century;[12] on the other hand, there could well be doubts as to whether this owed very much to the temperance movement. However, it should be pointed out that certain branches of the temperance movement did try actively to encourage people to drink non-alcoholic beverages as a substitute for liquor. The best example of this was the coffee public-house movement, which flourished from the 1870s until the end of the century. This was an attempt to wean the working classes away from drink by providing all the facilities of the public-house — games, entertainments, newspapers and so on — but selling coffee, tea, or cocoa instead of liquor. In the short term, the coffee public-houses were a limited success, and there existed several thousand of them in all parts of Britain during the 1880s and 1890s.[13] It is not possible to say how important this was in promoting the popularity of cocoa, but it clearly must have made some contribution. Ironically, this aspect of the temperance movement served also to perpetuate the obsolete technique and the adulterated product: aiming at the poorest stratum of society, and being essentially locally-based organisations, the coffee public-houses tended to provide an outlet for the cheap product of the small, local manufacturer. This is probably linked to another factor that might help us to understand the increasing level of consumption of cocoa products. Because of the various technological changes we have already described, there was a much purer, much less adulterated, product more generally available by the late nineteenth century. In two ways, this was important. For one thing, it set cocoa in sharp contrast to coffee, which continued to be a highly adulterated product right through into the twentieth century. In other words, there might well have been some substitution of cocoa for coffee.[14]

The second reason why the changing quality of cocoa might have been important concerns its changing image. To understand this more fully, we need to consider the sort of image cocoa had in the earlier period. One theme, above all, stands out: and that is the supposed medicinal and nutritive value of cocoa. The wholesome nature of cocoa as a beverage had been widely acclaimed since long before the nineteenth century. Probably, this was because of the genuinely exotic origins of the product, which is supposed to have featured prominently in the folklore of South American Indians, who regarded it as an elixir. The actual word cocoa is supposed to have its etymology in the language of the Aztecs; its scientific name was theobroma — food of the gods. The important thing for present purposes is that the belief continued into the nineteenth century that cocoa was, at the very least, a nourishing foodstuff, and, more than this, that it possessed medicinal properties. Indeed, the most conspicuous characteristic of contemporary advertisements was the emphasis on the medicinal value of the product. More reputable manufacturers made great use of recommendations by writers in *Lancet*, or the *British Medical Journal*. But it was the manufacturers of the old, adulterated cocoa who made the most extravagant claims for their product, usually with the support of some unknown and possibly fictitious medical authority. Take, for example, a product like Du Barry's Revalenta Arabica which claimed, in an advertisement quite typical of the 1870s, that it '... purifies and improves the blood, strengthens the stomach, nerves and muscles, removes all gastric or nervous irritability, ensures tranquil slumbers, absorbing and eliminating all acidity, feverishness, headaches, lassitude, constipation, dyspepsia, sleeplessness and low spirits'.[15] In fact, Du Barry's Revalenta Arabica was made in the East End of London by a firm with the not inappropriate name of Lye Brothers. It is possible to see the continuing emphasis on the medical properties of cocoa as a sort of *ex post* rationalisation: since the product must almost certainly have tasted like medicine, it was only logical to pretend that it had medicinal properties. The image of cocoa until as late as the 1870s was that of something which middle-class women took when they were suffering from constipation or some other indisposition. It is quite clear that, as a purer form of cocoa became more generally available, the emphasis in advertising changed: no longer did manufacturers emphasise medicinal properties so much; rather, they tended more and more to try to sell cocoa as a wholesome foodstuff which should form a regular item of diet. The importance of moving cocoa out of the medicine cabinet and into the larder is obvious. Levels of consumption were bound to rise if people were taking the beverage on a regular basis rather than just when they were feeling under the weather. It would seem that the late nineteenth century was a time when cocoa consumption was increasing not just because more people could afford it, but also because those who had always been able to afford it were beginning to purchase it more frequently.

It seems quite clear that an increasing proportion of cocoa products consumed in Britain was manufactured at home: in other words, imported cocoa was becoming less important. Van Houten, for example, were certainly nothing like the force in 1900 that they had been in the 1870s. In simple terms, the changing market situation elicited a response from British manufacturers. It would seem to be appropriate to conclude by looking at the response of British firms to the changing opportunities that occurred in the late nineteenth century — and by asking to what extent their experience throws light on any of the academic debates that surround these years. Perhaps the most obvious point to make is that this was not an industry characterised by entrepreneurial deficiencies. At the same time, there is a risk of going to the opposite extreme to that of writers like Aldcroft,[16] and categorising the name of Cadbury along with those of Lipton and Lever.[17] In fact, the success of firms like Cadbury and Rowntree does not reflect the achievements of a single, charismatic entrepreneur: rather it reflects the achievements of a series of men who were thorough, diligent, meticulous, and scrupulously honest — but in whom flair and imagination were not always the most conspicuous qualities. In fact, they worked within a code of business ethics which tended towards conservatism, and which certainly stopped short of pursuing ruthlessly the elimination of all rivals. Their reluctance to introduce alkaline cocoa, for example, shows that they were almost prepared to allow the precept that adulteration must be avoided at all costs to stand in the way of good business. However, once they were convinced that a particular line of business was worth pursuing — and it often took others to persuade them of this — then they pursued it successfully — with characteristic thoroughness and determination.

This industry is probably a good example of the sort of process that Professor Saul has analysed in parts of the engineering industry:[18] it is an industry which, in the long term, positively benefited from foreign competition. It learned the lessons and eventually took over markets in Britain which, arguably, had first been exploited by firms such as Van Houten or Menier. For reasons which have already been considered, there was from an early stage an awareness of what was going on abroad, a willingness to imitate anything that looked worth imitating. Both Rowntree's and Cadbury's were assiduous visitors to international exhibitions and trade fairs in various parts of Europe, always on the look-out for new ideas. This tends to reinforce the belief that we are here dealing with imitators rather than innovators; but, of course, imitators are often more successful than innovators.

There was a degree of organisation and co-operation within this industry far greater than the conventional textbook analysis of late nineteenth-century industry would suggest. Firms did communicate and meet with each other to discuss matters of common interest — resale price maintenance, foreign competition, raw material supply, trade marks, railway freight rates, and so on. Our view is not so much that this industry deviates from the norm in this respect; rather that the image of a vigorously competitive situation in British industry deviates somewhat from the reality.

There appears to be little evidence from this industry to support the view that entrepreneurs experienced difficulties in raising capital. The cocoa and chocolate industry was probably much in line with other consumer goods industries in that capital could always be obtained, usually from local sources. Moreover, the family firm could — and did —

grow into an organisation employing several thousand people. It also failed to display any reluctance to raise capital from outside the family, where circumstances dictated this — though control was always kept within the family by raising capital through the issue of non-voting preference shares.

In adapting to the changing circumstances of the late nineteenth century, the cocoa and chocolate industry kept abreast of the times, but was not in most respects a pioneer. It adjusted to changes in the use of advertising, but certainly did not lead the way. It adopted the corporate form, but no earlier than in other industries. It sought to develop overseas markets, particularly in the Empire; but, again, it was doing no more than joining a general trend. Perhaps the one area in which this industry can be said to have given a positive lead — albeit one which not many firms followed — was in the field of industrial relations. Rowntree's, Fry's and Cadbury's were all in the tradition of the paternalist employer — providing housing, education and welfare services for their employees. There can be little doubt that they did this for genuinely altruistic reasons, though there is no denying that this form of paternalism was not without its economic rewards in terms of stable labour relations, low rates of labour turnover, and so on.

What emerges out of all this seems to be something of an enigma. Here were firms and entrepreneurs which were undoubtedly successful, but which do not in all respects conform to the economic historian's ideal of the dynamic, growth-inducing entrepreneur. Certainly, they were players rather than gentlemen — to use a distinction drawn by one recent economic historian.[19] But they played the game according to their own peculiar set of rules, and were impatient of anyone who tried to disregard those rules. Perhaps what most distinguishes this industry from others is that, from an early stage of its development, it came to be dominated by a handful of large firms whose collective pressure could preserve the *status quo;* whereas, in many other industries, firms were neither strong enough nor sufficiently well-organised to ignore the determined newcomer who, like Lever in the soap industry, came along with a completely new set of rules.

Notes

1. This theme is considered more fully below, pp.79-83.
2. One estimate suggests that these three firms purchased between them up to two-thirds of the retained imports of raw cocoa into the United Kingdom.
3. The term adulterated is used to denote a product where starch has been added in order to counteract the fat content.
4. This comment occurs in private correspondence held in the firm's archives.
5. This theme is considered more fully below, pp.86-87.
6. The actual innovation is usually associated with the name of Peter, though it seems that other Swiss firms were quick to adopt the new technique.
7. For example, between 1900 and 1905, annual exports of chocolate from

Switzerland to Britain averaged nearly 13 million kilograms, compared with less than 3 million kilograms exported to Germany, the next most important market. These calculations are based on figures taken from *Gordian: Zeitschrift für die Schokoladenindustrie*, Hamburg.

8. *Le Chocolat Menier: une visite à l'usine de Noisiel*, n.d.
9. The main exception to this was the substantial re-export trade in cocoa beans. The extent of this is indicated by the gap between gross and net imports shown in Table I.
10. The following figures are cited by V.D. Wickizer, *Coffee, Cocoa and Tea: an Economic and Political Analysis*, 1951, p.264.

SHARE OF WORLD EXPORTS OF COCOA BEANS (%)

	1895	1909/13	1926/30
Latin America	86	62	34
Africa	10	35	64

11. See Table II above.
12. See, for example, figures quoted in Prest and Adams, op. cit.
13. Much information on the coffee public-house movement can be found in the newspaper of the organisation, *Coffee Public House News*, which appeared regularly between the 1870s and the 1890s.
14. Statistics quoted in Table II lend a certain amount of support to this suggestion.
15. The advertisement is one of a number held in the archives of Messrs. Cadbury Brothers.
16. D.H. Aldcroft, 'The Entrepreneur and the British Economy, 1870-1914', *Economic History Review*, 2nd ser. XVII (1964).
17. C.H. Wilson, 'Economy and Society in Late Victoria Britain', *Economic History Review*, XVIII (1965).
18. S.B. Saul, 'The American Impact on British Industry, 1895-1914', *Business History*, III (1960).
19. D.C. Coleman, 'Gentlemen and Players', *Economic History Review*, 2nd ser. XXVI (1973).

8 THE BRITISH TEA TRADE IN THE NINETEENTH CENTURY

P. MATHIAS

The tea trade underwent revolutionary expansion and structural change during the nineteenth century. These clearly documented aspects of the supply of tea imply equally revolutionary changes in patterns of demand and cultural norms lying behind dietary priorities, which are much less well known. This paper begins with an exposition of what happened in the tea trade and continues with less well-substantiated arguments which seek to explain the trends.

The graph shown in Fig. I and the statistics of imports reveal the pattern of supply and consumption very clearly, these figures being the retained imports of a commodity which could not be grown at home, and for which (during most of the nineteenth century) smuggling had ceased to be significant. They conceal, therefore, a considerable re-export trade from Britain which represented between one-fifth and one-sixth of the net import figures given here. In addition, if the story is seen as an astonishing record of expansion of production by the Indian and Ceylon tea industry, rather than a feat of consumption by British tea-drinkers, the direct exports from these countries to Australia, Russia, the United States and elsewhere have to be added.[1] Britain was taking about three-quarters of total exports from Ceylon, for example, at the end of the nineteenth century. The statistics tell their own story. For the first half of the century China was the sole source of supply of tea for this country, and trade was monopolised by the East India Company until 1834. Although total retained imports rose on trend (from 23.73m. lbs. in 1807 to 36.68m. in 1841) they were increasing with population expansion rather than through any increase in consumption *per capita*, which stagnated at a level between 1.25 lbs. and 1.50 lbs. per annum during this period. The break in trend came during the 1840s when cumulative expansion of retained imports for domestic consumption began at a quite new pace, explained by the continuing rise in numbers but now also buttressed by a steady increase in consumption *per capita*, which rose from 1.90 lbs. in 1851 to 6.50 lbs. *per capita* in 1911. Consumption *per capita* doubled in the twenty years between 1841 and 1861; it doubled again between 1861 and 1871. Although subsequent rates of growth were not as dramatic in percentage terms, the increments in tonnage were more formidable: the sustained nature of the expansion represented a fundamental change in the drinking habits of the nation.

The figures also clearly reveal that increments to sustain the demand for increased supplies of tea came not from China but from India after

Figure I: *British Tea Trade in the Nineteenth Century*

Year	Net imports (M. lbs.)	Consumption per cap. (lbs.)	Rate of Duty
1801	23.73	1.50	30% *ad valorem*
1811	22.46	1.25	96% *ad valorem*
1821	26.75	1.25	96% *ad valorem*
1831	30.00	1.25	96% *ad valorem*
1841	36.68	1.38	2s. 1d. per lb. (1841)
1851	53.95	1.90	2s. 1d. per lb.
1861	77.94	2.75	1s. 5d. per lb. (1861)
1871	135.53	3.90	6d. per lb. (1863)
1881	160.22	4.62	6d. per lb.
1891	202.40	5.38	4d. per lb. (1890)
1901	258.85	6.13	4d. per lb.
1911	295.26	6.50	5d. per lb. (1908-9)

Sources of Tea Imports to UK (%)

	China	India	Ceylon
1866	95.6	4.4	–
1876	82.0	18.0	–
1886	58.1	37.9	4.0
1896	10.9	54.0	35.1
1906	7.0	58.9	34.1

Sources: *Parl. Papers* 1894, LXVIII (321); 1911, LXXXVII (521); D.M. Forrest, *Tea for the British*, 1973, p.285; P. Griffiths, *History of the Indian Tea Industry*, 1967, p.125; P. Mathias, *Retailing Revolution*, 1967, p.30-31; G.R. Porter, *Progress of the Nation*, 1912 edn., pp.444-50.

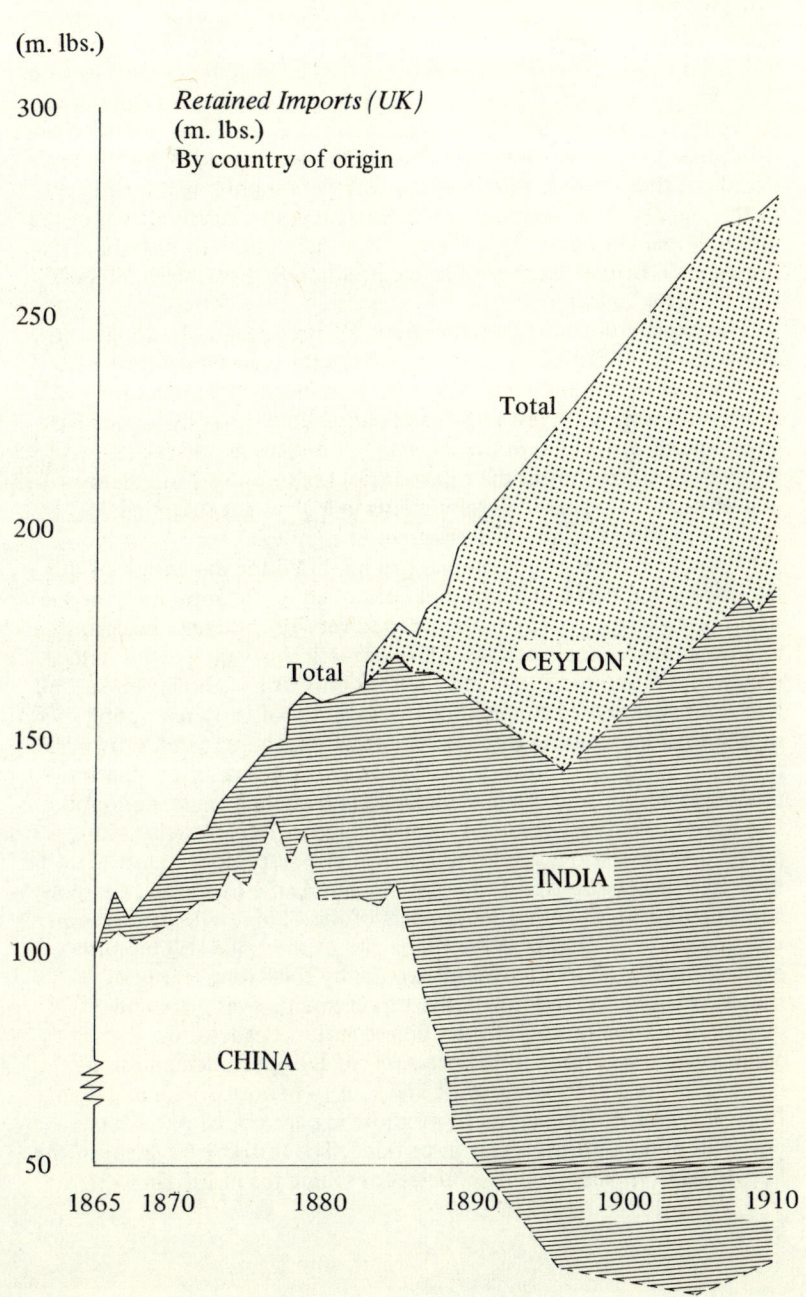

1860, and were increasingly supplemented by Ceylon teas after 1883. China sustained the increase to a level of *c.*100–125m. lbs. per annum but not beyond that, so that supplies from China between 1870 and 1885 became fairly unresponsive to increasing demand; they were being maintained in the aggregate but represented a steadily falling share of the teas being sold in the British market. After 1885, tea imported from China fell away very sharply in absolute quantities from *c.* 100m. lbs. to 25m. lbs., which then made up less than ten per cent of the rapidly expanding total British market. Indian teas, on the other hand, rose to occupy over half of total tea sales in the UK by the last decade of the century, when Ceylon teas were supplying a further third of the market. Thus, expansion was integral with a restructuring of the international tea trade, from China to the sub-continent of India, from 'foreign' to 'British' enterprise in the production areas, from 'green' teas to 'black' teas.

The explanations for these dramatic changes have to be sought in many places: in China, India and Ceylon, with their contrasting experiences in responding to the expansion in world demand for tea; in alterations in tax levels on tea and competing drinks by successive governments in Britain; in the changes in purchasing power of British families; in alterations in their patterns of consumption and dietary conventions; in dramatic developments in high street shopping. We begin with the situation in the sources of supply.

A double barrier of constraints had inhibited the expansion of the tea trade when based in China and controlled by the monopoly of the East India Company. The Company had very restrictive policies and arrangements for such a trade. All their tactical advantages lay with a policy of restriction. They held auctions only at East India House, and were more concerned to maintain prices and profits by restricting supply than maximising total income from expanding sales. Provincial merchant groups put pressure on Parliament to break this China trade monopoly by the East India Company (as its Indian trade monopoly had been broken in 1813) and this was done in 1834 – with great public demonstrations celebrating the end of despotic restraint with the first 'free' tea auctions in 1834-5 at Mincing Lane, Liverpool, Glasgow and Bristol. But, as with other aspects of the China trade, it was soon revealed that constraints at the China end of the trade still inhibited expansion. Monopoly control of exports by the 'Hong' cartel of Chinese Merchants, very restrictive arrangements over price and quantity, and the refusal of the Chinese authorities to allow the commercial opportunities and pressures of European demand to be made effective in the tea-growing areas, or to permit British merchants to organise, or British capital to promote expansion, all put a very powerful brake on the extension of trade. The restrictive system of the East India Company, and its policies for selling tea in Britain were revealed to have been a logical counterpart to a restrictive system in China.

One of the ironies of this situation was that the solution for alternative supplies had been conceived and contrived by the East India Company itself in the hey-day of its China monopoly, although this initiative was slow in bearing fruit. In 1828 the Governor General, Lord William Bentinck, received a detailed memorandum from a Mr. Walker proposing that tea should be developed as a commercial crop in Assam because of the continuing uncertainties of commerce with China and the social imperative tea now commanded in Britain. 'It has become a luxury to all,' ran the text, 'and almost a portion of food to the common people, who in some districts drink it three or four times a day. Its use is so intermingled with our habits and customs that it would not easily be dispensed with.'[2]

Sir Joseph Banks had proposed this for India as far back as 1784; but it was following Walker's petition that a committee of Calcutta merchants and officials (including the director of the Botanic Garden at Calcutta, Dr. Wallich), was set up by Bentinck to draw up proposals. They could draw on the results of much private initiative by Wallich in propagating Chinese tea seeds and plants and scouring Assam and neighbouring areas for wild, indigenous teas. The first Indian plantation teas were auctioned at East India House in 1839.

A similar sequence then ensued in Ceylon. Private efforts were made to indigenise tea plants there as far back as 1816. In 1839 the Royal Botanic Gardens near Kandy propagated seeds from the Calcutta Botanic Garden, sent by Wallich, and commercial cultivation began with an effective informal collaboration of civil servants, professional botanists and commercial planters – in the Ceylon case, oddly, German Jews from Frankfurt-on-Main, Gabriel and M. B. Worms, who were related to the Rothschilds. By the 1860s a Planters Association had been formed (but coffee planting was the boom crop, with 176,000 acres under coffee in 1869, and 1 m. cwts. shipped in 1870. Fungus attacks in the coffee crop in 1870 and following years precipitated a switch to tea, although 19 acres had been laid down to tea in the first large-scale planting in 1867 – a very long diffusion time from the initial experiments of thirty, or more, years before. The original objective was to produce for the local national market, but the first consignment was supposedly sent to London in 1873 and the first auctions began in Ceylon in 1883.[3]

The subsequent sequences are shown in Fig. I, with a steep rise from the 1m. lb. level after 1883.

The astonishing capacity of India and Ceylon to respond to rising world demand for tea is to be explained by many factors. No institutional constraints stood in the way of expansion. The Indian and Ceylon administration was favourable (Calcutta thought settlement and plantations would consolidate a border zone politically), and actively helpful in the development stage. A 'plantation' commercial base in coffee had already developed. Labour was plentiful or could be organised from large-scale Tamil immigration to the Ceylon gardens without official objections. Such a work-force was efficiently organised and very cheap. Above all British capital, merchant firms and enterprise could sponsor the projects, which were potentially highly profitable in commercial terms, and take charge of the new industry. A considerable amount of new technology was quickly developed, with mechanised rolling, aerial ropeways and large-scale organisation of drying and packing. Very sophisticated merchanting and commercial organisations were established in India and Ceylon. The trade became an extension of the most efficient commercial organisation of commodity markets in the world, then being established in Britain under the impetus of a free-trade policy which was making the United Kingdom the largest importer of food and raw materials in the international economy.

This very efficient deployment of merchanting methods which established the matrix for expansion had direct links with the London market and retailing interests in England. And here the new standards of competitiveness being set by the multiple shops in high streets in all the main urban centres of the country have to be considered.[4] This was another important pre-condition for revolutionising the tea trade, once the constraints on supply had been resolved. Thomas Lipton bought over 7000 acres of tea plantation in Ceylon following a whirlwind three-week visit in June 1890. He advertised this new commitment aggressively (as always) 'direct from the tea garden to the tea pot' with a Tamil girl on all the tea-packets. Integration from retailing to plantation ownership was not characteristic of the organisation of the trade, however, and remained quite unrepresentative even for Lipton's trade (apart from the 'advertising' imperative). Almost all plantations, and the tea trade in general, were British-controlled; but not by retailers owning shops and integrating back to their sources of supply. Only a very small proportion of the tea sold by Lipton (which grew into a world-wide business, apart from selling over the counters of his shops in Britain) came from his own estates: tea auctions in Colombo, Calcutta and London were his main recourse for acquiring supplies – with an efficient buying, warehousing and shipping organisation. A presence in tea production, however, was a useful peg for publicity and, more importantly, gave him a presence in production to judge costs and quality independently. Brooke Bond developed an equivalent world-wide trade, with a presence in the tea states, without owning shops; and this was the truly representative pattern.

Just as the great expansion of the trade involved structural change on the supply side, so equally there was change in techniques of selling.

Most of the increments in sales were through the medium of new-style mass retailing by multiple shops and co-operative stores in the mass markets of urban England, and a rising proportion of these sales were in pre-packaged tea. Most aspects of this style of trading developed in the greatest contrast to the conventions of the middle-class grocer.

The pattern of the new mass retailing was integral with tea-selling, but had been set slightly earlier with other commodities, particularly ham and bacon. The characteristics were the same: the shops sold a very few lines in a mass trade, offering good quality with elemental facilities at very low margins, taking advantage of economies of scale and the rapidly falling price available from imported commodities, advertising, aggressively seeking to tap the extra purchasing power flowing to the urban working classes. Sugar, cheese, ham, bacon, butter, eggs and margarine underwent this commercial transformation, as well as the tea trade. Most of Lipton's shops sold six or seven commodities only at this period. Some of the larger chains even had the word 'tea' in their title, in recognition of their degree of specialisation. This was the case with the 'International Tea Stores', and most of the Home and Colonial Stores shops were blazoned as specialist 'Tea Stores' (with a small minority of larger shops in main city centres with a wider range of lines). Collectively the new retailing turned the older style of trade on its head: this had been characterised by general grocers and provision merchants offering a very diversified and large number of lines, in middle-class areas, for principally middle-class customers. Retailing businesses were individual family-owned shops for the most part, with assistants dispensing specialised skills in preparing, mixing and making up portions at the time of the sale. The commercial characteristics of this style of trade meant wide margins, high rates of profits, high unit costs, and low stock-turn. The pay-off in prices brought by the new style retailing of multiple shops was dramatic: low production costs, economies of scale in processing, merchanting, and distribution, falling transport costs, a more efficient distributive system aimed at a growing mass market and a policy of taking low rates of profit on bulk turnover became translated into falling prices. This was the essential characteristic of the multiples and co-operative stores; it provided the leverage for all their advertising; the main motivation for the mass of their customers, and the principal objective of their entire commercial system.

Retail prices of tea (Hyson) which had stood between 13*s.* and 14*s.* per lb. between 1803 and the 1830s fell to 5*s.* to 8*s.* per lb. in 1841 with the change in duty. The change from a duty rate of 96 per cent *ad valorem* to 2*s.* 1*d.* per lb. in 1841 effectively halved the tax while prices *net* of duty rose between 1840 and 1870, this being more than compensated by the fall in duty rates from 2*s.* 1*d.* per lb. to 6*d.* per lb. When Lipton entered the trade in 1890 he found prices of green teas at 3*s.* to 4*s.* per lb. in the family grocers and, with the other multiples, undercut at a level of 1s. 2d. – 1s. 9d. per lb. In 1900-1905 prices were still ranging from 1s. 4d. – 1s. 8d. per lb. in the multiples. Thus the duty changes had the greatest impact upon this decline in price until 1870; but thereafter increasing efficiencies in the production of tea in India and Ceylon, and increased competition and lower cost distributions in the UK market proved the major influences of change.

The context of demand after 1850, as we have emphasised, was also particularly favourable. Population of the UK rose from 27m. to 45m. between 1851 and 1911: that of Great Britain (the heart of these developments) doubled from 20m. to 40m. in the same period, always growing by more than 10 per cent per decade. Money wages doubled between 1850 and 1910 (increasing by one-third between 1880 and 1914), while prices fell by 40 per cent between 1870 and 1895 (particularly occasioned by the fall in the prices of imported foodstuffs – including tea). Thus the increasing extent of demand, brought by a rising population, was augmented by a widening of demand *per capita* occasioned by rising real wages.

Into this pattern we have to fit the trends of competing commodities. In a sense, the black Indian and Ceylon teas *were* a different commodity from the original product – the China green and Hyson teas. They proved much more robust than green teas for processing and handling; they were 'stronger' in infusing and more economical in use per unit of weight. But competing and complementary products apart from tea provide critical comparisons.

It is important to see that the tea boom was not to be explained, until after 1899, by a relative or complementary decline in the consumption of beer or spirits.

There was a short-term decline in beer and spirits sales *per capita* between 1875-6 and 1886-7, but then strong recovery took place again until 1899-1900. From 1900-14 consumption per head of spirits and beer again declined. Thus, in two separate periods, 1875-86 and 1900-14, tea gained by substitution; but tea consumption also advanced as rapidly during other periods when the consumption *per capita* of potentially competing drinks was also rising.[5]

The figures at troughs and peaks are:

Table I: *UK* per capita *consumption of spirits and beer*

1875	1.3 galls. spirits (peak)	
1876		34.4 galls. beer (peak)
1886		27.9 galls. beer (trough)
1887	0.93 galls. spirits (trough)	
....		
1899		32.5 galls. beer (peak)
1900	1.12 galls. spirits (peak)	

For this reason I do not believe that certain other changes, such as the falling ratio of licensed premises to population or the temperance movement had much influence in the long term: the public-houses and gin palaces got larger, even if their numbers fell *per capita* of the population, and the temperance movement waxed at those times and in those regions where the sale of alcoholic drinks was booming.

Of greater significance may have been the relative movement in the prices of beer (with other alcoholic drinks) and tea in influencing the distribution of rising effective demand between the alcoholic drinks and tea. Whereas the range of prices of tea fell dramatically between 1840 and 1890, beer prices remained very steady over the whole period after 1830, the effect of switching tax from malt to beer, and some subsequent increases in tax being mainly taken out in varying the strength of the beer (specific gravities, then as now, remaining the brewer's secret). What these relative shifts embody, however, is evidently a considerable change in the social role of alcoholic drinks, a much more mysterious business, and the changing social and cultural role of the public-house. In earlier periods, beer-drinking fulfilled several social and cultural roles, not being differentiated as a necessity, nor as a target for surplus spending. Beer was drunk in the family, and as a mealtime drink, as well as being the focus for the main leisure/relaxation activity in public-houses. Much greater discrimination developed between these roles in the course of the nineteenth century. Also with tea. Tea in the eighteenth century — and even into the nineteenth with commentators such as William Cobbett — had been commonly condemned as an extravagant luxury leading the nation down the path of degeneracy, perverting the poor, psychologically and even physiologically. The condemnation was cast in similar terms to that by which gin in the eighteenth century and subsequently beer, smoking cannabis and other pleasures of the rich have been successively condemned in the nineteenth and twentieth centuries as they pass down the social structure to become necessities of the poor. The social role of tea-drinking became transformed from indulgence in an expensive luxury to that of a daily necessity as the habit descended the social pyramid. Differentiation then occurred on both sides between tea and beer, with beer sales increasingly being for non-family, non-meal, social, pleasure and surplus-income drinking, while tea sales supplied the basic domestic, home family brew. This represents, of course, a crude caricature of what remained, and remains, a complicated picture. But profound restructuring undoubtedly occurred in both trades during this period, as other restructurings have occurred subsequently.

As David Allen's investigations into *British Tastes* made clear for our own times, dietary patterns have great complementarities and interrelatedness. There are essential complementarities between foodstuffs: obvious links between bread, butter (or margarine) and jam;

fish and chips and the like; or between foodstuffs and drinks — as between tea and sugar; but less obviously between the food and drink commodities and other aspects of life-style. Consumption patterns are influenced by such things as whether pleasure and leisure are taken at home, or whether a cooked tea is taken or not. Such considerations take us into the most mysterious unplumbed depths of social and cultural history — which suggests that it is the appropriate point for an economic historian's text to stop and discussion by a social nutritionist to begin.

Notes

1. G. R. Porter, *Progress of the Nation,* 1912 edn., pp.444-50; B. R. Mitchell, *Abstract of British Historical Statistics,* 1962, pp.298-9, 307-8; D.M. Forrest, *A Hundred Years of Ceylon Tea 1867-1967,* 1967, pp.288, 290-1.
2. Quoted by P. Griffiths, *History of the Indian Tea Industry,* 1967, p.37.
3. See D.M. Forrest, op. cit; D.M. Forrest, *Tea for the British,* 1973; P. Griffiths, op. cit.
4. For an extended treatment of tea retailing in Britain, and Lipton's world-wide trade in tea, see P. Mathias, *Retailing Revolution,* 1967, Chs. 6 and 16.
5. G.B. Wilson, *Alcohol and the Nation,* 1940.

PART TWO: FACTORS INFLUENCING CONSUMPTION

9 THE AGRICULTURAL LABOURER'S STANDARD OF LIVING IN KENT 1790-1840

T.L. RICHARDSON

In recent years the revival of interest in the standard of living controversy has produced very little new statistical evidence on wages and prices.[1] To a large extent the lack of a consensus of agreement on what happened to working-class living standards has been due to a dearth of reliable wage and price data covering the period 1790-1840.[2] Indeed, our knowledge of commodity prices, and especially of the commodities normally purchased by the labouring classes in this period is extremely limited and what is known about prices in areas outside of London is negligible.[3] Most of our knowledge about the cost of living in the late eighteenth and early nineteenth centuries is restricted to a few price series derived from various London institutions.[4] Although these sources provide a useful general guide to the cost of living their main limitation is that they apply only to London and cannot be used to make generalisations about other areas. During the eighteenth century, for example, there were several regional market areas in existence and each one had its own price history and its own set of price relationships.[5] Until these price relationships are investigated and analysed it cannot be assumed that prices were uniformly the same over a wide area and that the cost of living in London was representative of the cost of living in the country at large.[6] A further weakness with this kind of evidence is the difficulty of knowing to what extent contract prices can be used to measure changes in the cost of living. Until more is known about the relationship between contract prices and retail prices any conclusions regarding the standard of living, which are based upon this kind of evidence, must be regarded as speculative. Ideally, what is needed is a number of indexes, each derived from a different area, or region, relating to a specific occupational group, and containing in their composition the prices of the kinds of commodities most normally consumed by that social group.

An important source of primary evidence which would fulfil this *desiderata,* and which has been largely ignored by historians of the past,[7] is to be found in the Provisions Accounts of parish poorhouses and work houses.[8] Before the passing of the 1834 Poor Law Amendment Act each individual parish was responsible for the maintenance of its poor and it therefore became necessary for parish overseers to make regular purchases of a wide range of groceries and provisions for the sustenance of the poor and needy. These provisions were usually of a similar kind and quality to those found in the household diets of the labouring classes living in the area and included such items as bread, flour, meat (beef, mutton, and pork), cheese, butter, tea, sugar, candles, soap, and shoes.[9] All these commodities were usually supplied by shopkeepers who traded in the area and it was the general custom to award the contract to the suppliers who tendered the lowest price and offered the highest discounts. At Sandhurst in May 1820, for example, a local miller offered to supply the workhouse with flour at 1*d*. a gallon less than the prevailing retail price. At the same time a butcher offered to supply the workhouse with meat 'at one-half penny per pound under his ready money price'. Other shopkeepers agreed to supply groceries and provisions at prices 5 per cent less than their retail prices.[10] In St. Margaret's parish, Rochester, a local baker agreed to supply the workhouse with best white bread for 2*d*. a gallon less than the prevailing London Assize price in 1812.[11] At that time the price of the gallon loaf in London was 3*s*. 4*d*.[12] Similar offers to these were made in November 1813 and April 1814 when gallon loaves were offered at 2½*d*. and 3*d*. below the prevailing London Assize price; the price of the gallon loaf in London being 2*s*. 4*d*. and 2*s*. 1½*d*. respectively at that time.[13] Similar examples to these are to be found in the parish records of other counties[14] and serve to confirm the impression that workhouse provisions' contract prices were, on average, five to ten per cent lower than prevailing market prices.[15] This situation changed, however, after 1834 when groups of twenty or more individual parishes were grouped into Poor Law Unions. This administrative change meant that substantial quantities of provisions were required for the maintenance of large numbers of paupers. As these contracts were highly lucrative to suppliers, the Poor Law Unions were able to obtain their provisions at prices which were on average 18 per cent less than the prices paid by individual parishes.[16]

The importance of this kind of evidence is that it provides a valuable insight into the relationship between contract prices and retail prices and provides several continuous runs of prices of the kinds of commodities normally consumed by the labouring classes in the area.[17] This statistical evidence is invaluable for constructing a regional cost of living index, especially as contract prices were fairly sensitive to changes in market prices.[18] Contract prices were usually fixed for short periods of one to three months and were constantly adjusted at the renewal of the contract to even out any possible price discrepancies and to ensure that no side to the contract suffered a financial loss. The significance of this practice was that contract prices were fairly responsive to short-run price changes in local markets and therefore tended to reflect quite closely fluctuations in the prevailing cost of living.[19]

The statistical evidence on commodity prices (and agricultural wages) in Kent is fairly abundant and for this study a range of prices has been derived from the Provisions Accounts of eight parishes and three Poor Law Unions.[20] All these parishes are evenly dispersed over the central area of the county and an average of the prices of the various commodities in these areas has been used to formulate, in Laspeyres form, a cost of living index.[21] The 'basket' of commodities which comprise the index contains six main categories of expenditure[22] — food and drink, cottage rent,[23] fuel,[24] candles, soap, and shoes[25] — and these have been weighted in accordance with the amount of expenditure agricultural labourers laid out on these items in their household budgets:[26]

Table I: *Distribution of Household Expenditure (%)*

Food and Drink	67.7
Cottage Rent	8.8
Fuel	5.4
Clothing	10.2
Shoes	1.7
Candles	1.5
Soap	1.5
Miscellaneous	3.2
	100.0

It is evident from an analysis of these budgets that as much as two-thirds of the labourers' total household expenditure was spent on food and drink. The provision of three basic necessities of life — food, shelter, and warmth — absorbed over 90 per cent of the labourers' income, leaving a slender margin over for all their other domestic needs.[27] The various consumables in the food and drink category have been weighted in a similar way according to the amount of expenditure spent on them in these budgets.[28] As the distribution of household expenditure of food and drink changed from one year to another the weights in the index have been adjusted accordingly:

Table II: *Distribution of Household Expenditure on Food and Drink*

	1793[29]	1812[30]	1814	1821	1835[31]	1837	1838
	%	%	%	%	%	%	%
Bread/Flour	48.0	74.2	55.8	64.2	49.0	46.1	57.1
Meat	26.2	6.0	10.0	9.3	16.2	16.2	15.1
Cheese	10.0	9.0	13.4	10.4	8.5	12.2	5.3
Butter	8.0	6.0	10.2	7.8	11.3	13.5	11.8
Sugar	5.3	2.0	4.7	3.0	5.8	7.0	5.0
Tea	2.5	2.2	4.0	3.4	5.0	5.0	5.7
	100.0	99.4	98.1	98.1	95.8	100.0	100.0

These budgets throw considerable light upon the way expenditure patterns changed under the impact of wartime inflation and post-war deflation. With the outbreak of war with France, for example, acute shortages of foodstuffs led to a rise in the prices of bread, meat, and sugar by 167 per cent, 100 per cent, and 41 per cent respectively by 1812. These increases were accompanied by marked shifts in the distribution of expenditure on these commodities. The most notable 'Giffen effect' which resulted from these price increases was a 26 per cent increase in expenditure on bread, a 20 per cent decrease in the amount spent on meat, and a halving of expenditure on sugar. As expenditure on bread absorbed such a high proportion of the labourers' expenditure on food and drink, the 167 per cent increase in its price between 1790 and 1812 had such a devastating effect[32] upon the labourers' real incomes that they were forced to reallocate their expenditure and introduce a degree of substitution into their diets.[33] It was a well-known phenomenon to contemporary observers that when real incomes fell[34] due to a rise in the general cost of living the labouring classes were obliged to reduce their consumption of 'luxury' goods such as meat and sugar, whose demand was relatively elastic, in order to afford the basic necessities of life such as bread, whose demand was inelastic.[35] As one observer of this practice noted, 'I believe it has always been found that among labourers the first diminution takes place in tea, meat, sugar, and things of that nature, much rather than in bread'.[36]

Falling prices at the end of the war, and during the post-war agricultural depression, brought about a partial reversal of the wartime pattern of expenditure on food and drink. Between 1812, the peak year for prices during the war, and 1823, the nadir in the post-war price depression, the price of bread more than halved itself,[37] thus making possible a reallocation of expenditure in favour of 'luxury' commodities and a more varied diet. It is evident from the figures of household expenditure between 1814 and 1838 that the marked fall in the price of bread was accompanied by a proportionate reduction in the amount spent on it in the family budgets. As expenditure on bread fell to a level which was about the same as in the 1790s, this was offset by an increase in household expenditure on commodities such as meat and tea.[38]

The history of the cost of living in Kent between 1790 and 1840 falls into three sub-periods; a period of soaring inflation between 1794 and 1812, a period of pronounced deflation (except for 1817) between 1812 and 1823, and a period of price recovery from 1823 to the early 1830s. The major peaks in the cost of living, which occurred in 1795, 1800-1, and 1812, were closely associated with violent increases in food prices which, because of the relatively high weight attached to food and drink in the index, tended to determine the rate of oscillation in the all-items index. Given the inelasticity of agricultural supply in the short-run, the main causes of inflation were a succession of disastrous harvest failures and a fall in foreign imports of corn.[39] The prices of imported tropical products such as tea and sugar were artificially raised by the imposition of exorbitant customs and excise duties,[40] whilst domestic prices of bread, meat, cheese, butter, leather and tallow doubled by 1812. The combined effect of these developments was to increase the cost of living in Kent by 120 per cent by 1812.

The ending of the war with France, coupled with improvements in domestic harvests,[41] improved the general agricultural supply situation between 1812 and 1823 and brought about a marked diminution in the cost of living through a substantial fall in food prices. Except for a sharp increase in 1817, due to a poor harvest, the prices of all the principal commodities in the food and drink category were halved between 1812 and 1823 and the cost of living index fell to a level which was a mere 7 per cent higher than in 1790. This sequence of events was somewhat reversed after the agricultural depression of the early 1820s by a series of poor harvests[42] which lifted the general level of prices to a point which was about 30 per cent higher than the 1790 position by the early 1830s.

The standard of living controversy is primarily concerned with long-run changes in the purchasing power of wages. In this study the statistical evidence on agricultural wages has been derived from the Cobham Hall Estate Labour Accounts.[43] This evidence, which covers an unbroken run of fifty years, relates to the average weekly earnings of agricultural labourers employed on the estate and forms the basis from which an index of real wages has been calculated.[44]

It is evident from an examination of the cost of living curve and wage earnings curve in Figure I that a fairly close degree of correlation existed between the two, with the former series tending to outstrip the latter on a number of occasions. Indeed, the fact that increases in agricultural labourers' earnings tended to lag behind marked fluctuations in the cost of living meant that the purchasing power of wages was substantially reduced for a period of about twenty-six years. The most serious reductions occurred during the Napoleonic War, and in 1817, where a dramatic increase in the cost of living, coupled with a lag in agricultural wages, plunged the index of real wages to a level 14 to 22 per cent below the level prevailing in 1790.

In 1815 the era of agricultural prosperity and full employment was reversed and replaced by a post-war era of deflation, agricultural distress, and widespread rural unemployment and underemployment.[45] In such uncertain times as these, the agricultural labourers' standard of living was primarily determined by whether or not he could obtain regular employment. For those labourers in regular employment at Cobham, the post-war deflation brought no improvement in the standard of living as agricultural earnings were deflated by a corresponding amount, thus continuing to depress the index of real wages until the mid-1820s. Indeed, the first real improvement in the index occurred from 1825 onwards, though this was only a mere 5 per cent betterment on the 1790 position.

A 5 per cent improvement in real wages after a wait of thirty-five years was but a modest gain for labourers who were in regular employment. For labourers who were only able to obtain employment at irregular intervals their standard of living situation must have been lamentable. Indeed, one of the outstanding characteristics of the post-war labour market in Kent was the surfeit of rural labour. In certain years the numbers of out-of-work labourers reached alarmingly high levels as many farmers, in seeking to cut their costs and minimise their losses, drastically reduced their labour force during the winter quarter of the year. From the evidence collated in the Board of Agriculture's survey, *The Agricultural State of the Kingdom, 1816*, it is evident that in some parts of Kent as much as a quarter to a third of the rural labour force were out of work.[46] According to a correspondent from Maidstone, in west Kent, the farmers there were 'obliged to part with perhaps a third of their labourers' and that the labourers were 'very distressed for want of employment'.[47] Another witness commented,

> Nothing can be more wretched than the state of the labouring poor, ... One third, I should think, were out of employ, and a portion of the remainder working at a price which is insufficient to maintain their families.[48]

The numbers of agricultural labourers without work in Kent remained at a high level throughout the 1820s and 1830s and provided a background of poverty and social tension which eventually culminated in the 'Swing' riots of 1830.[49] Most Wealden parishes, for example, had a surplus labour problem during this period. Out of a total population of 21,719 living in sixteen parishes 8,263 were paupers, and a further 682 were unable to obtain employment at any time of the year.[50] William Cobbett, as he journeyed through the corn-growing areas of east Kent in 1823 commented, 'It is impossible to have an idea of anything more miserable than the state of the labourers in this part of the country.'[51]

In view of the existence of high levels of cyclical and seasonal unemployment it is evident that a large proportion of the agricultural labour force stood to suffer a substantial reduction in its standard of living due to no fault of its own. Prolonged bouts of unemployment during a downturn in the rural trade cycle brought the labourers' annual average earnings down with a run and plunged as many as a

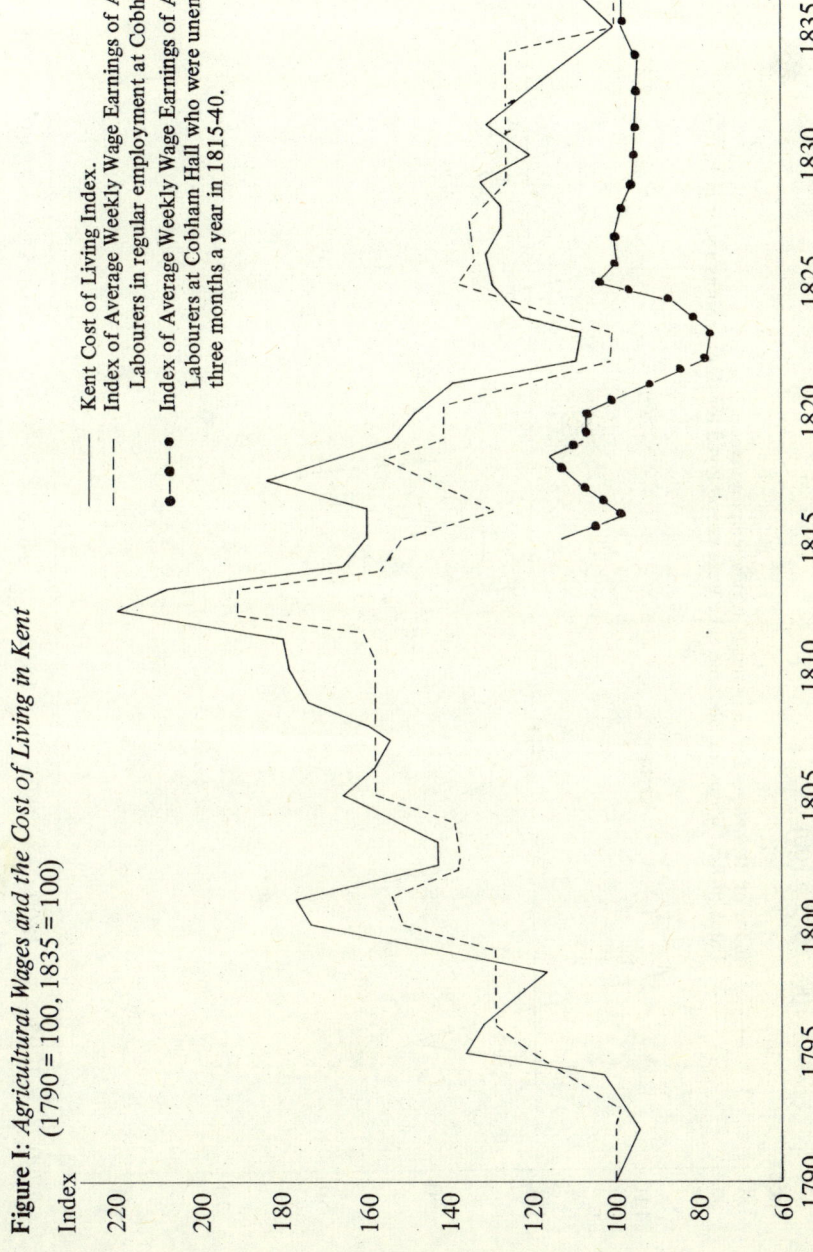

Figure I: *Agricultural Wages and the Cost of Living in Kent*
(1790 = 100, 1835 = 100)

——— Kent Cost of Living Index.
– – – Index of Average Weekly Wage Earnings of Agricultural Labourers in regular employment at Cobham Hall.
●–●–● Index of Average Weekly Wage Earnings of Agricultural Labourers at Cobham Hall who were unemployed for three months a year in 1815-40.

Figure II: *Index of Agricultural Labourer's Real Wages in Kent*
(1790 = 100, 1835 = 100)

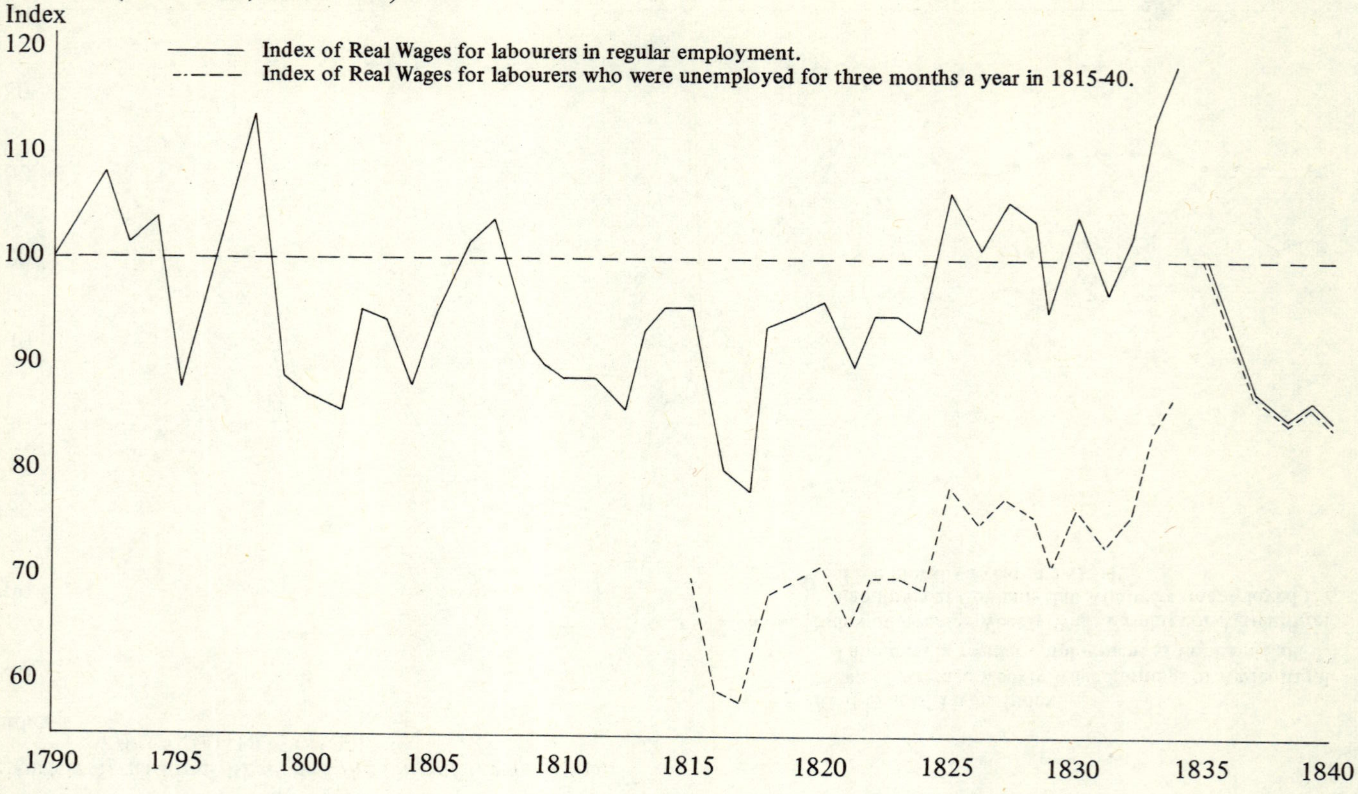

Index

——— Index of Real Wages for labourers in regular employment.
- - - - Index of Real Wages for labourers who were unemployed for three months a year in 1815-40.

third or more of the agricultural labour force into a state of penury. Any conclusions regarding the standard of living in Kent must therefore be weighted in accordance with the size of this element. As a first step it has been shown that in an ideal situation agricultural labourers who were able to obtain regular employment and maximise their earnings at Cobham Hall did not achieve any appreciable improvement in their standard of living until after 1825. Prior to that date the index of real wages was almost continually depressed below its 1790 position. If the labourers' standard of living showed little improvement under the somewhat favourable circumstances of full employment, then the condition of that sizeable proportion of the rural labour force who were unable to find work during the winter quarter of the year must have been desperate. If, then, some allowance is made for a loss of earnings due to winter unemployment, as in Figures I and II, a more balanced picture begins to emerge which shows a catastrophic fall in real wages for almost the whole of the period 1790-1840. Somewhere between this lower limit and the upper limit of full employment, lay the bulk of the agricultural labour force and therein a substantial part of the answer to the standard of living question.

Notes

1. The leading contributors to the debate are: T.S. Ashton, 'The Standard of Life of the Workers in England, 1790-1830', *The Journal of Economic History,* IX (1949); E.J. Hobsbawm, 'The British Standard of Living, 1790-1850', *The Economic History Review,* 2nd ser. X, 1 (1957); S. Pollard, 'Investment, Consumption and the Industrial Revolution, *EHR,* 2nd ser. XI, 2 (1958); R.M. Hartwell, 'Interpretations of the Industrial Revolution in England', *JEH,* XIX (1959); A.J. Taylor, 'Progress and Poverty in Britain 1750-1850', *History,* XLV (1960); R.M. Hartwell, 'The Rising Standard of Living in England, 1800-1850', *EHR,* 2nd ser. XIII, 3 (1961); E.J. Hobsbawm, 'The Standard of Living during the Industrial Revolution: A Discussion', and R.M. Hartwell, 'The Standard of Living', *EHR,* 2nd ser. XVI, 2 (1965); J.E. Williams, 'The British Standard of Living, 1750-1850', *EHR,* 2nd ser. XIX, 3 (1966). See also E.P. Thompson, *The Making of the English Working Class,* London, 1964. Other contributors are mentioned below.
2. A further difficulty is that different contributors refer to different time periods. T.S. Ashton wrote of the period 1790-1830, E.J. Hobsbawm 1790-1850, A.J. Taylor 1750-1850, R.M. Hartwell 1800-1850, S. Pollard 1745-55 to 1840-50, and J.E. Williams 1750-1850. Similarly, these writers have written about the 'British standard of living' and the 'English standard of living'. Much of the debate's inconclusiveness can be attributed to the absence of agreement on whose standard of living is being considered and in what time period.
3. B.R. Mitchell and P. Deane, *Abstract of British Historical Statistics,* Cambridge, 1962, pp.338-40, 466. See also G.H. Wood, 'The Investigation of Retail Prices', *JRSS,* LXV (1902), p.685. Some notable exceptions are: R.S. Neale, 'The Standard of Living, 1780-1844: A Regional and Class Study', *EHR,* 2nd ser. XIX, 3 (1966); G.J. Barnsby, 'The Standard of Living in the Black Country during the Nineteenth Century', *EHR,* 2nd ser. XXIV, 2 (1971); T.R. Gourvish,

'The Cost of Living in the Early Nineteenth Century', *EHR*, 2nd ser. XXV, 1 (1972). See also M.W. Flinn, 'Trends in Real Wages, 1750-1850', *EHR*, 2nd ser. XXVII, 3 (1974).
4. N.J. Silberling, 'British Prices and Business Cycles, 1779-1850', *Review of Economic Statistics*, V, Supplement II (1923); E.B. Schumpeter, 'English Prices and Public Finance, 1660-1822', *RES*, XX (1938), p.32; E.W. Gilboy, 'The Cost of Living and Real Wages in Eighteenth Century England', *RES*, XVIII (1936), p.136; A.D. Gayer, W.W. Rostow and A.J. Schwartz, *The Growth and Fluctuation of the British Economy, 1750-1850*, Oxford, 1953, pp.475-6; E.H. Phelps Brown and S.V. Hopkins, 'Seven Centuries of the Prices of Consumables compared with Builders' Wage-Rates', *Economica*, XXIII (1956).
5. Thorold Rogers recognised six price regions: (1) the Metropolitan or Thames region; (2) the Eastern Counties; (3) the Midland Counties lying between the Trent and the Thames; (4) the Southern region lying between Kent and Devon; (5) the South-West region; (6) the Northern region to the north of the Trent. J.E.T. Rogers, *A History of Agriculture and Prices in England*, Oxford, 1887, V, pp.239-40. See also P. Deane and W.A. Cole, *British Economic Growth 1688-1959*, Cambridge, 1967, p.12.
6. By the late eighteenth century there is some evidence to show that under the impact of improved communications local market autonomies were breaking down and regional price differences were being smoothed out and moved into line with one another as large quantities of wheat were moved from areas of surplus to areas of scarcity. C.W.J. Granger and C.M. Elliott, 'A Fresh Look at Wheat Prices and Markets in the Eighteenth Century', *EHR*, 2nd ser. XX, 2 (1967), pp.257-65.
7. According to one historian this neglect was due to the fact that 'the economic historian's hostility to the use of prices paid by public institutions in constructing a cost of living index has persisted because of a failure to appreciate the high correlation between retail and contract prices'. W. Woodruff, 'Capitalism and the Historians: A Contribution to the Discussion on the Industrial Revolution in England', *Journal of Economic History*, XVI (1956), p.5.
8. These are usually located in County Record Offices.
9. As most Poor Law officials were concerned to keep expenditure on poor relief to a minimum they tended to apply the Poor Law Commissioners' recommendation that workhouse diets were 'in no case to exceed, in quantity and quality of food, the ordinary diet of the able-bodied labourers living within the same district'. *First Annual Report of the Poor Law Commissioners for England and Wales*, Parl. Papers 1835, XXXV, London, 1835, p.98.
10. Kent Record Office, P 321/8/1. Sandhurst Parish Vestry Minutes.
11. KRO, P/R/305/12/13. St. Margaret's Parish, Rochester.
12. *The Maidstone Journal*, August 1812.
13. ibid., November 1813, April 1814.
14. Essex Record Office, D/P 118/18/2. Cranham Parish Overseer's Accounts. J.E. Oxley, *Barking Vestry Minutes*, Colchester, 1955, p.244.
15. In the 1790s the Rev. J. Howlett of Dunmow noted that workhouses in Suffolk and Essex obtained their provisions at prices which were 10 per cent lower than prevailing market prices. *Annals of Agriculture*, XXV (1796), p.602. See also A. Young, *The Farmer's Tour Through the East of England*, London, 1771, II, pp.185-6, and Lord Beveridge, *Prices and Wages in England*, London, 1939, pp.312-57.
16. *First Annual Report of the Poor Law Commissioners*, op. cit., p.98. Owing to the administrative changes in the Poor Law in 1834 and its effect upon discount rates two base years, 1790 and 1835, have been used in calculating the cost of living index.

17. As this study is primarily concerned with the rate at which prices increased or decreased after a given base year, rather than the actual level of prices, the contract prices used in this study have not been adjusted to take account of discount rates.
18. In Pembury parish the vestry officers accepted a local tender to supply the workhouse with provisions as the price was 'fair . . . according to the present state of the market'. KRO P286/8/1, Pembury Parish Vestry Minutes 1820-55. If the market price increased after the contract had been agreed upon, suppliers sometimes refused to honour the contract until the buyer had paid them a higher price. ERO D/P 115/8/1-2. Hornchurch Parish Vestry Minutes 1826-30.
19. Long-term contracts lasting for six months or more tended to be 'sticky' and lagged behind changes in market prices. Long-term contracts also disguised qualitative changes in commodities which sometimes took place to offset an increase in market prices. Schumpeter, op. cit., p.33.
20. KRO: P 78/18/1-6, 66-82. Charing Parish Workhouse Provisions Accounts. P 243/12/7-21. West Malling Parish Workhouse Provisions Accounts. PR 305/12/6-15. St. Margaret's Parish (Rochester) Workhouse Provisions Accounts. P 244/18/1-3. Lenham Parish Workhouse Provisions Accounts. P 100/12/17. Cranbrook Parish Workhouse Provisions Accounts. P 406/12/17. Wrotham Parish Workhouse Provisions Accounts. P 184/12/8-10. Hever Parish Workhouse Provisions Accounts. P 347/8/1. Staplehurst Parish Workhouse Provisions Accounts. G/Me/AMI. Malling Poor Law Union Minute Book. G/Ee/AMI. Elham Poor Law Union Minute Book. G/AW/AMI. West Ashford Poor Law Union Minute Book. Bread prices have been derived from the Faversham and Queenborough Assize of Bread, and from the sources listed above. KRO Fa/Aa 61. Faversham Borough Records. The Assize of Bread. KRO Qb/AA. Queenborough Borough Records. The Assize of Bread.
21. The prices used in the index are annual averages of monthly prices.
22. It has been necessary to omit clothing from the index as it has been impossible to locate any evidence on the prices of garments in Poor Law records.
23. One of the most intractable problems encountered in this study has been the difficulty of measuring changes in cottage rents. No continuous series of rents for various types of dwellings seem to exist and it has therefore been necessary to assume that cottage rents remained constant between 1790-1840. This assumption will tend to understate, rather than overstate, the actual rise in the cost of living as there is some evidence to suggest that cottage rents doubled in this period. See, for example, J. Marriage, *Letters on the Distressed State of the Agricultural Labourers,* Chelmsford, 1832, II, pp.5, 17-18; J. Caird, *English Agriculture in 1850-51,* London, 1852, p.474; J. Glyde, *Suffolk in the Nineteenth Century,* London, 1856, p.358.
24. Coal has been used to represent fuel in this study as prices of other fuels were not available. Coal was the most common fuel purchased by the workhouses and although it is probable that the labouring classes burnt wood, peat, turf, or animal dung on their fires there is insufficient evidence to quantify these fuels and incorporate them in the index.
25. Agricultural labourers usually wore boots rather than shoes. Boot prices, however were not available but as both commodities were manufactured from the same raw material it is reasonable to expect that their prices would fluctuate by a similar proportionate amount from a given base year.
26. D. Davies, *The Case of Labourers in Husbandry Stated and Considered,* London, 1795, pp.180-3. The weights attached to each category are expressed as a proportion of total household expenditure. The Miscellaneous category, which includes such imponderables as medicine and lying-in, has been omitted owing to a lack of specific information.

27. It is interesting to note that in the second half of the nineteenth century agricultural labourers spent about 67 per cent of their income on food and drink, 10 per cent on fuel and light, 12 per cent on clothes, and 10 per cent on cottage rent. H.J. Little, 'The Agricultural Labourer', *JRAS*, 2nd ser., XIV (1878), p.777; *Royal Commission on Labour. The Agricultural Labourer, England*, I, Parl. Papers 1893-4, XXXV, p.129; *Second Report on the Wages and Employment of Agricultural Labourers in the United Kingdom*, Parl. Papers 1905, XCVII, 1913, p.230. In 1966 the distribution of household expenditure in Britain was as follows: food, drink and tobacco 38.2 per cent, fuel, light, and power 6.2 per cent, clothing and footwear 9.3 per cent, housing 10 per cent, soap and matches 1.1 per cent. *Ministry of Labour Family Expenditure Survey. 1966 Report*, London, 1967, pp.20-23.

28. Owing to a lack of information on milk, beer and potatoes, it has not been possible to include these items in the index. According to the opinions of contemporary observers, however, the main beverage of Kentish labourers was tea because milk was 'very scarce' and they could 'seldom . . . afford to drink beer'. F.M. Eden, *The State of the Poor*, A.G.L. Rogers (ed.), London, 1928, pp.210-11; *Annals of Agriculture*, XXIV (1795), pp 86-7, 175, 180. See also Davies, op. cit., pp.38-9, and *Reports of Special Assistant Poor Law Commissioners on the Employment of Women and Children in Agriculture*, Parl. Papers 1843, XII, 1843, p.183.

29. Davies, op. cit., pp.180-3. Davies derived these budgets from counties adjacent to Kent.

30. KRO P 244/8/2; Marden Parish Vestry Minutes 1814-23. The budgets for 1812, 1814 and 1821 relate to six families, composed of 12 adults and 31 children, and were collected by parish officials who were investigating into the amount and cost of provisions required to support these families 'as given by themselves'.

31. F. Purdy, 'On the Earnings of Agricultural Labourers in England and Wales', *JRSS*, XXIV (1861), p.363. These budgets relate to seven families comprising 14 adults and 29 children.

32. Rising prices, caused by acute food shortages during the Napoleonic War, became a focus of popular discontent in Kent which sometimes erupted into riots and public demonstrations. *The Maidstone Journal*, 17 February 1795, p.4; *Annals of Agriculture*, XXXIV (1800), p.113, 601-7.

33. When wheat was in short supply the government continually urged the labouring classes to reduce their consumption of wheaten bread and eat bread made from mixed grains such as barley, oats, and rye. E. Melling, *Kentish Sources: IV. The Poor*, Maidstone, 1964, pp.152-4. The labouring classes, however, sometimes refused to substitute brown bread for white on the grounds that they had 'lost their rye teeth' and that it 'disordered their bowels'. Eden, op. cit., pp.105, 209. Davies, op. cit., p.32. Potatoes, rice and herrings were often recommended to the poor as suitable alternatives to wheaten bread and there is some evidence to show in contemporary journals such as the *Annals of Agriculture* that some such substitution took place, though it is not possible to quantify the extent to which this happened and incorporate it into a cost of living index. See also R.N. Salaman, *The History and Social Influence of the Potato*, Cambridge, 1949.

34. Between 1790 and 1812 the index of real wages fell by 14 per cent.

35. T. Tooke, *Thoughts and Details on High and Low Prices of the Thirty Years from 1793 to 1822*, London, 1824, p.164. See also J.C. McKenzie, 'Past Dietary Trends as an Aid to Prediction', in T.C. Barker, J.C. McKenzie and J. Yudkin (eds.), *Our Changing Fare*, London, 1966.

36. *Report from the Select Committee on the Depressed State of Agriculture*,

Parl. Papers 1821, IX, p.118. Eden, who visited Kent during the 1790s, made a reference to the reduction in meat consumption amongst the poorer classes in the country. Eden, op. cit., p.208.

37. Between 1812 and 1823 the average annual weekly price of the quartern loaf in Kent fell from 1s. 6d. to 7d. The quartern loaf weighed 4 lb. 5½ oz.

38. The proportion of expenditure on meat during the 1820s and 1830s did not increase to the level it held in the 1790s, probably because the price of bread did not fall to its pre-war level again but remained at about a 30 per cent higher level.

39. The 1799 wheat crop was estimated to be deficient by one-quarter to one-third its normal yield. *Annals of Agriculture*, XXXIV (1800), pp.601, 635. See also T. Tooke and W. Newmarch, *A History of Prices, 1792-1856;* M. Olsen, *The Economics of the Wartime Shortage*, Durham, USA, 1963; E.L. Jones, *Seasons and Prices*, London, 1964.

40. In 1790 the duty on a pound of tea stood at 12½ per cent of its value. This was increased with the outbreak of war with France to 30 per cent in 1797, and to 65 per cent and 96 per cent respectively in 1803 and 1807. The Budget of 1819 retained the duty of 96 per cent on tea costing under 2s. 0d. a pound, but added 4 per cent on tea costing more than this, thus bringing the duty to a 100 per cent. This increase brought the average amount of duty paid on a pound of tea to 2s. 11d. which represented a threefold increase on the duty levied in 1784. From 1820 to 1823 the duty remained at 2s. 9½d. a pound and thereafter progressively declined to reach 2s. 1¾d. a pound in 1840.
In 1790 the duty on sugar was 12s. 3d. per hundredweight. It increased to 15s. 0d. in 1791-6 and, as the war progressed, to 20s. 0d. in 1800-04, and to 27s. 0d. in 1805-12. In 1813-15 the duty rose to 30s. 0d. a hundredweight, doubling the duty which prevailed in 1791, and up to 1823 fluctuated between 27s. 0d. and 30s. 0d. a hundredweight. The sugar duty was reduced to 24s. 0d. in 1830, and it remained at that level until 1840 when a further 5 per cent was added. See Tooke, op. cit., pp.46-9, 58-61; G.R. Porter, *The Progress of the Nation*, F.W. Hurst (ed.), London, 1912, p.444; *Report on Wholesale and Retail Prices in the United Kingdom in 1902*, Parl. Papers 1903, LXVIII, p.176; L.M. Brown, *The Board of Trade and the Free Trade Movement, 1830-42*, Oxford, 1958, pp.36, 149.

41. The 1820 harvest was so abundant that its effect upon market prices lasted for two or three years. Tooke and Newmarch, II, op. cit., p.82.

42. The harvests of 1823, 1824 and 1829 were deficient in quality and quantity. Tooke and Newmarch, op. cit., pp.132-4; *The Maidstone Journal*, 1 September 1829, p.4.

43. KRO U565/A9a-54a, A314. Lord Darnley. Cobham Hall Estate Labour Accounts.

44. The index of real wages has been calculated by dividing the wage earnings index by the cost of living index. It will be appreciated that real wages are not the sole measure of the labourers' standard of living. Besides receiving cash wages some labourers were also paid in kind (harvest victuals, farm produce below its market price; free cottages, allotments, and fuel) either as a supplement to low wages or in lieu of cash wages. The task of balancing the beneficial effects of these non-monetary allowances against the deleterious effects, whilst taking into account the fact that these customs did not prevail in all areas of the country and were already disappearing by the early 1800s in the areas where they did prevail, involves innumerable practical and methodological problems which are not easily reduced to a statistical form. For these reasons the labourers'

wage earnings have been taken as the yardstick by which his standard of living may be judged to have improved or deteriorated.

45. N. Gash, 'Rural Unemployment, 1815-34', *EHR*, VI, 1 (1935); E.L. Jones, 'The Agricultural Labour Market in England, 1793-1872', *EHR*, XVII, 2 (1964).
46. Board of Agriculture, *The Agricultural State of the Kingdom, 1816*, 1816; Reprinted London, 1970, pp.123-40.
47. ibid.
48. ibid., p.136.
49. T.L. Richardson, 'The Agricultural Labourers' Riots in Kent in 1830', *Cantium. Kent Local History* (Winter, 1974), pp.73-5.
50. *Report from the Select Committee on Emigration from the United Kingdom*, Parl. Papers 1826, IV, 1, pp.135-8.
51. W. Cobbett, *Rural Rides*, G. Woodcock (ed.), London, 1967, p.206.

10 DRINK AND WORKING-CLASS LIVING STANDARDS IN BRITAIN, 1870-1914[1]

A.E. DINGLE

It is generally accepted that the period covered by the 'great depression' witnessed a more rapid and sustained increase in real wages for the bulk of the working class than had hitherto been achieved. But it would be dangerous to assume too readily that this indicated a proportional rise in working-class living standards in any wider sense. In 1899 Seebohm Rowntree found 18 per cent of all wage-earners in York living in 'secondary poverty', due to the nutritionally unwise allocation of an income which, if well spent, would have been sufficient to provide for 'merely physical efficiency'.[2] A recent survey of working-class dietary has highlighted 'the apparent paradox between the rise in real wages and the low standards of nutrition and health' at the end of the nineteenth century.[3] Many contemporary middle-class observers of working-class life resolved this paradox by emphasising that the working man was his own worst enemy due to his indulgence in forms of expenditure which were economically damaging and socially undesirable. It was expenditure on 'intoxicating liquors' which was regarded above all others as the major obstacle to improvement. Social historians have since tended to accept the validity of this claim.[4] What follows is an examination of the changing level of drink consumption and expenditure between 1870 and 1914, and an attempt to assess the extent to which this expenditure inhibited any improvement in working-class living standards which might be expected to follow from rising real wages.

Estimates of Consumption

Fig. I shows the level of consumption per head of the two main alcoholic drinks, beer and spirits; expenditure on the two accounted for over 90 per cent of the total drink bill between 1870 and 1914, with beer accounting for just under 60 per cent on average and spirits just over 30 per cent. In general, the period 1870-1914 probably saw a rise to the peak level of nineteenth-century consumption,[5] and the beginning of a gradual and temporarily interrupted long-term decline. Beer did not however fall to the levels prevailing in the 1840s until after the First World War. For spirits the long-term trend before 1900 is less clear but from 1900 onwards there was a decline in consumption levels below those which had prevailed throughout the nineteenth century. Between 1870 and 1914 the two items exhibit very similar variations. There is a rapid rise to a peak in 1875-6 of over 34 gallons per head for beer, and nearly one and a half gallons per head in the case of spirits.

Figure I: *UK Drink Consumption per Head, 1850-1914*

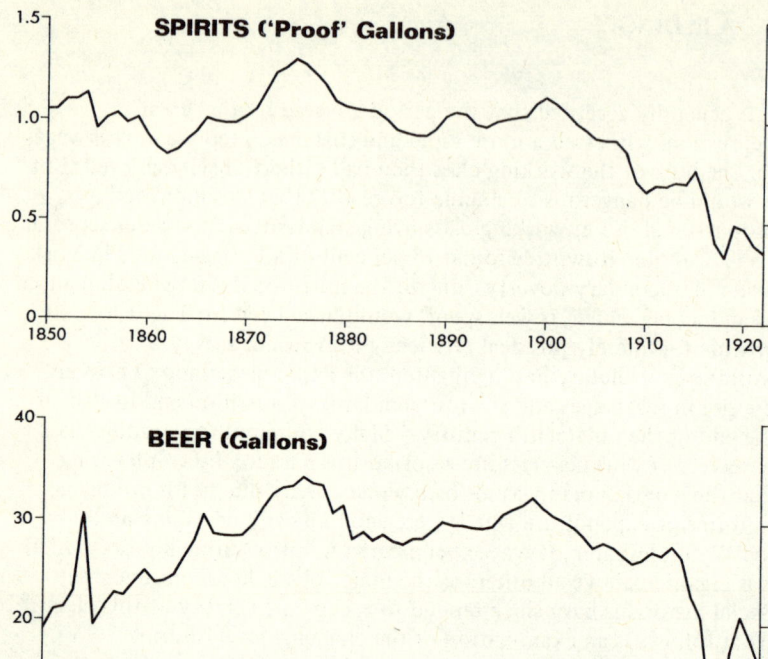

Source: G.B. Wilson, *Alcohol and the Nation,* 1940, pp.332-3.

There was an equally rapid fall to 1881 for beer and 1879 for spirits. This was followed by a period of little change in consumption levels, contrasting with the more marked fluctuations which had preceded it. Beer remained at between 28 and 30 gallons per head, and spirits between 0.93 and 1.07 gallons. A lesser peak was then reached in 1899-1900, followed by a decline which was distorted by the war, but continued after it. Although the pattern of change for the two items was similar, the magnitude of the change was not. For example, beer consumption rose by 20.3 per cent between 1870 and the peak of 1876, while spirits rose by 28.8 per cent between 1870 and 1875.

These statistical data suffer from weakness.[6] Until 1880 beer consumption figures are derived indirectly from the quantity of malt and sugar used in commercial brewing. Home brewing for private consumption is not included; this activity was declining considerably, however, and from 1870 the figures given are unlikely greatly to understate the level of consumption. After 1880 the basis of taxation was the 'standard barrel' with a fixed official specific gravity (1057° from 1880 to 1889 and 1055° from 1889 to 1933). Beer was, however, often brewed at a lower specific gravity, so the number of barrels for sale, or 'bulk barrels', exceeded the number of 'standard barrels'. After 1900, increases in beer and licence duties were passed on to the consumer in the form of beer of lower specific gravities (and hence lower alcoholic content), while maintaining constant price levels. But once again this is unlikely greatly to understate the level of consumption or significantly alter the trends observed in Fig. I.

A further weakness of the statistics is that they give no indication of regional variations in the level or habits of drink consumption. England accounted for the bulk of beer drunk, also gin and rum, while whisky was drunk mainly in Scotland and Ireland.[7] Perhaps more importantly, there appear to have been marked variations in the drinking habits of different areas. Statistics of drunkenness are dubious indicators of the level of drink consumption, reliant as they are on the degree of police stringency,[8] but they suggest that the major ports were the most drunken places in the country, followed by mining towns, London, industrial towns, resort towns, and lastly agricultural counties.[9] Certainly contemporaries considered drunkenness to be a largely urban problem.

Figures for drink consumption per head give little indication of the actual level of consumption of those who drank. But any attempt to be more precise can be little more than a 'guestimate', given the lack of data on the number of non-drinkers. In 1871 Leone Levi argued that 56 per cent of the population consumed alcohol in one form or another. Joseph Rowntree and Arthur Sherwell accepted this (as did the 'trade'), and refined it still further by suggesting that children under 15 years of age did not drink and that on average women drank half as much as men. This gave a consumption of 73 gallons of beer, 2.4 gallons of spirits, and just under a gallon of wine for each male drinker in 1898.[10] But in assessing the economic effect of drink consumption it is expenditure levels rather than consumption levels which are more significant. In order to gauge the impact of drink expenditure on the family budget, the fact that wife and children are abstainers is irrelevant as they are still affected to the extent that some part of the family budget is spent on drink by the wage-earner. Of greater value would be data on the number of adult male abstainers who were heads of households, but even the temperance movement, with its penchant for collecting statistics, failed on this score.[11]

Between 1870 and 1914 the price of alcoholic drinks remained remarkably constant, with beer at 2½d. a pint, spirits averaging 3s. 4d. a pint (proof), and wine averaging 3d. a pint.[12] This being so, the changing level of drink consumption over this period also represents the pattern of expenditure on drink per head. Expenditure per head per year moved up from £2.19s.6½d. in 1850 to a peak of £4.9s. in 1876, then fell back to below £3.15s. during the eighties and early nineties. A lesser peak of just under £4 was reached in 1899. About one-fifth of this expenditure went in taxation. The drink trade was an important source of government revenue, with taxes on drink and licence duties combined accounting for about one-third of total governmental tax revenue between 1850 and 1900, reaching as high as 43.4 per cent of the total in 1879-80.[13]

Personal expenditure on drink can give only an imperfect indication of the economic effect of drink consumption unless it can be related in some way to income. Fig. II attempts to do this at a national level by showing expenditure on drink as a percentage of total consumer expenditure on goods and services, at current prices. From a peak of over 15 per cent in 1876, drink expenditure levels out at between 12 and 13 per cent from the early 1880s to the end of the century; it then falls considerably to 1914. An independent spot check on Fig. II is provided by the investigations of the British Association for the Advancement of Science in 1881. The 'Committee ... on the Present Appropriation of Wages'[14] found that out of a total daily expenditure on goods and services of 16.6d. per head (9.6d. daily going on food and drink), 2.3d. was spent on alcoholic drink, amounting to about 14 per cent of total expenditure. Drink was the largest single item, followed by meat at 1.9d. per day accounting for 11.4 per cent of the total, and bread at 1.4d. accounting for 8.8 per cent of total expenditure.

The conclusions of contemporaries as to the proportion of working-class incomes spent on drink were highly impressionistic. This is hardly surprising given the difficulties in obtaining reliable information,[15] but these estimates were all higher than the national averages indicated in Fig. II. Charles Booth suggested it was common for one-quarter of working-class earnings to be spent on drink as did George Sims, while Seebohm Rowntree accepted one-sixth as a reasonable estimate for York. A recent investigator has concluded that 'many families must have spent a third, and some one half or more, of all their income on drink'.[16] In regard to the allocation of the total drink bill, Levi considered that the working class purchased 75 per cent of all beer and spirits, and 10 per cent of all wine sold.[17] While not relying too much on the accuracy of this evidence it does appear reasonable to assume that the working man spent a larger proportion of his income on drink than did the more affluent; and that the major part, perhaps two-thirds to three-quarters, of all spending on drink

Figure II: *UK Expenditure on Drink as a Percentage of Total Consumer Expenditure on Goods and Services at Current Prices*

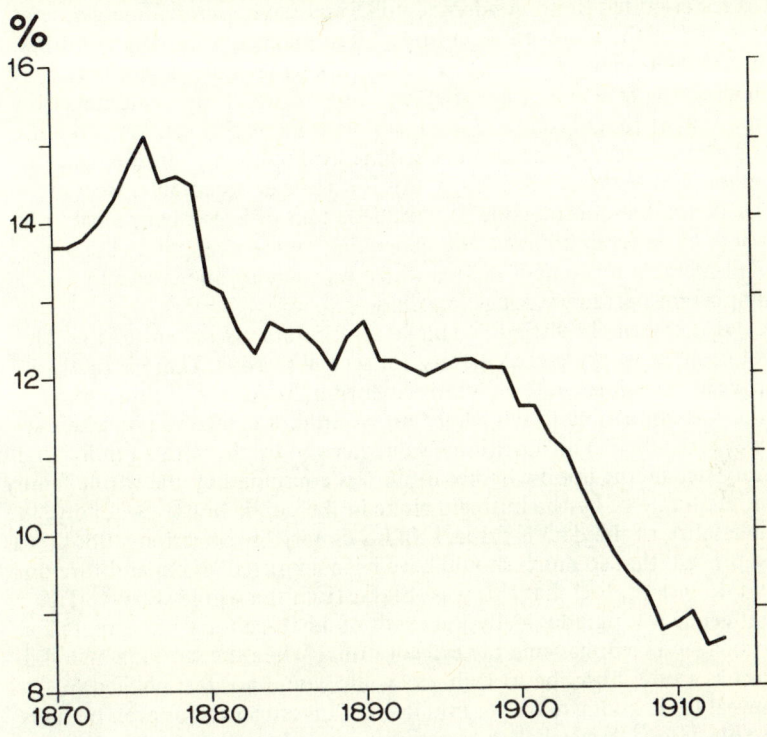

Sources: Total consumer expenditure: J.B. Jefferys and D. Walters, 'National Income and Expenditure of the United Kingdom 1870-1952', *Income and Wealth*, ser. V, p.27. Expenditure on drink: A.R. Prest, *Consumers' Expenditure in the United Kingdom 1900-1919,* Cambridge, 1954, pp.75, 85.

came out of working-class pockets. Therefore Fig. II probably somewhat understates the proportion of working-class purchasing power absorbed by drink.

The Energy Value of Alcohol in the Diet

Less attention has been paid to living standards in the last third of the nineteenth century than during the period of early industrialisation; there is less at stake and the issue is less in doubt. Even after allowance has been made for their deficiencies, the available real wage series show an unmistakable upward trend. The optimistic conclusions drawn from these have been based on the assumption that, 'with adequate incomes people buy foods which are nutritionally desirable'.[28] This generally seems to have been the case, but there were the important exceptions of roller-milled flour, condensed milk, and unvitaminised margarine at the end of the nineteenth century.[19] Temperance reformers put drink in the same category. The view that drink was wholly deleterious, having no place in a proper diet, was one for which the temperance movement fought long and hard, and with increasing success, from the 1870s onwards, against entrenched medical opinion.[20] In the light of modern nutritional knowledge, this is no longer acceptable. Beer in particular has considerable food value, a pint of beer having a calorific value of between 200 and 400 depending on the strength of the brew,[21] considerably more than the tea which was playing an increasingly important part in working-class diet.

It is extremely difficult to make an accurate assessment of the role of drink in working-class dietary for several reasons. There is firstly a paucity of evidence; few dietaries mention drink, and of those which do, it is impossible to tell what type of drink was involved or where it was consumed. The nutritional value derived by the whole family would vary depending upon whether drink was consumed by the whole family in the home or by the husband alone in the public house. Secondly, the reliability of the data is suspect. In his dietary investigations, Booth was surprised 'that so much should have been admitted' as expenditure on drink, but implied that this was still far from the whole story.[22] This reticence was paradoxically the result of a half-century of temperance propaganda emphasising the evils of drink. While the working man did not as a rule subscribe to such a view, he would not feel obliged to reveal his drinking habits to middle-class investigators, or even perhaps to his wife.[23] Nevertheless, in families where income was either inadequate or barely adequate to provide for the maintenance of 'merely physical efficiency', drink could be purchased only at the expense of essential foodstuffs. But drink provided an escape not only from a barren environment but also, up to the 1880s at least, from a monotonous diet.

A crude assessment of the implications of this choice can be made on the basis of the budgetary investigations of Miss W.A. MacKenzie.[24] She constructed hypothetical budgets for representative groups of the population in 1860, 1880, and 1914. The object was:

> to supply the most common articles of food in such quantities as the total available supply, and the wage received, would allow, subject to the custom of the time, as far as this could be ascertained from descriptions of diet, etc. The calorie value of the diet as thus determined has been calculated with the object of seeing how far such a diet supplied the necessary nourishment.[25]

Two standards were adopted, a minimum one of 3,000 calories per man per day, or 81,000 calories per standard family per week (standard family = man, wife, and three schoolchildren, or 3.87 'men'), and a more liberal one of 3,500 calories per man per day, or 95,000 calories per standard family per week. Alcoholic drink was not included in the budgets.

The median family at the top of the unskilled work-force in 1880 earned a weekly wage of 26s. 6d. of which 16s. 0¾d. was spent on food and drink. This yielded 94,100 kilocalories, each penny expended giving 488 kcals. Beer on the other hand, on the assumption of an alcoholic content of 5 per cent, and a price of 2½d. per pint, yielded 115 kcals for each penny spent.[26] If it is further assumed that 14 per cent of total income was spent on drink (the average national figure)[27] this would give a weekly expenditure of 3s. 8½d. If this amount were spent entirely on beer, it would yield 5,140 kcals. If however this sum had been spent so as to obtain the average value of the alcohol-free food intake of 488 kcals per penny spent, it would have yielded 21,720 kcals. So for the median family this expenditure on drink represented a net weekly loss of 16,580 kcals, reducing the total intake from 94,100 to 75,520 kcals and below minimum requirements. The standards set need not be taken too seriously; it is arguable that they are perhaps too high. The important point is that spending on drink reduced the calorific intake of the family by 17.6 per cent.

This example probably understates the calorific loss experienced by working-class families due to expenditure on drink, for several reasons. Firstly, as already mentioned, the proportion of working-class incomes spent on drink is likely to have been higher than the national average shown in Fig. II. Secondly, the calorific intake derived from alcohol is unlikely to have been equally distributed over the whole family. Much was consumed in the public house and would therefore benefit only the husband and to a lesser extent perhaps his wife. The calorific intake of the children is likely to have been much lower than the example indicates. Finally, a penny spent on beer provided more than twice as many calories as a penny spent on spirits. Therefore by assuming only beer was consumed, the resultant calorific loss has been minimised.[28]

It is clear that while drink was a significant source of energy, it was not a cheap source. Therefore for those with incomes little above the 'poverty line' expenditure on drink could push them below it, by reducing their calorific intake to less than minimum requirements, and below what could have been achieved if cheaper sources of calorific energy had been chosen. This confirms the findings of Booth and Rowntree, that expenditure on drink was a cause of 'secondary poverty'; for Rowntree it was the 'predominant factor' in accounting for the 18 per cent of wage-earners living in secondary poverty in York in 1899.[29]

However, if a similar calculation is made for Miss MacKenzie's median family in 1914, a somewhat different picture emerges. Fig. II indicates that a much smaller proportion of a larger weekly wage was being spent on drink: 8.6 per cent of a weekly wage of 35s. 6d. But in monetary terms this represented only a small drop in expenditure from 3s. 8½d. in 1880 to 3s. in 1914. Each penny spent in the alcohol-free diet yielded a calorific value of 395. This was a considerably lower figure than in 1880 due to a shift in consumption patterns from cheap carbohydrates to more expensive proteins as a source of energy. It meant that the calorific differential between a penny spent on beer or on other foodstuffs was being narrowed. The tendency for drink to depress living standards was therefore being lessened. The weekly calorific intake of 106,900 in an alcohol-free diet was reduced to 96,392 with the addition of beer. This was still above the higher of the two standards adopted and represented a reduction in weekly calorific intake of only 9.6 per cent. The changes evident between 1880 and 1914 suggest the need for an examination of some of the determinants of the changing level of drink consumption shown in Fig. I, in order to throw light on why the adverse impact of drink on nutritional standards was being lessened.

Changing Patterns of Consumption

Contemporaries explained changes in the level of drink consumption per head in terms of a wide range of determinants; climatic variations, types and hours of work, the number of retail outlets in relation to population, the availability of alternative recreational facilities, and the growth in temperance sentiment all had their advocates. But it was widely accepted that the main determinant of variations in consumption over time was the level of wages and commercial prosperity. It was in these terms that the peak level of consumption in 1875-6 was explained.[30] More sophisticated statistical analysis has confirmed the positive correlation between wages and drink consumption, the closest correlation being observed after a one-year lag, and for spirits to a greater extent than for beer.[31] But while this explains short-term fluctuations, by itself it does not adequately account for either the magnitude of consumption levels reached in the mid-1870s or the subsequent long-term trend of virtual stagnation, and after 1900, decline, despite continued rises in both real and money wages.

The rise in consumption in the 1870s confirmed the worst fears of temperance reformers, i.e. that rising incomes were not effectively generating an improved standard of living because of the consequent increase in drink expenditure. While real wages rose 16.1 per cent between 1870 and 1876, beer consumption rose 20.3 per cent and spirits consumption was up 25.7 per cent. In beer consumption the peak appears to be the logical climax to rising incomes, and consequent increases in consumption, from the 1850s onwards. For spirits, however, the peak constitutes a clear break from an otherwise almost unchanging level between 1850 and 1900.

Contemporaries certainly considered that the 1870s were exceptional: 'The deterioration which had taken place in the working classes had been deplorable. The rise of wages coming upon a class of men ill-prepared for it, was a positive evil of the highest degree.' It was felt that 'the period of transition from low to high wages, and from incessant toil to comparative leisure, must be one of peril to the masses', until the 'moral condition' of the working class was improved.[32] It has recently been suggested that a change in consumption habits in response to rising wages may not come smoothly and automatically in the first instance: 'a profound sociological problem is lost sight of, if our minds run simply in terms of varying injections of money into the family purse.'[33] It is argued that a majority of the work-force were enjoying a significant increase in purchasing power for the first time, and this was being imposed upon consumption patterns which were both narrow and conventionalised. Without a background of rational budgetary knowledge upon which to draw, increased purchasing power was likely to be squandered on drink and other luxuries once traditional needs had been met. The situation was exacerbated in mill and mining towns, with their solidly working-class populations, where the absence of middle-class example gave rise to 'a fixed frame of convention to which all tended to conform and which was hostile to improvement'.[34] During the boom of the early 1870s, 'miners indulging in Champagne wine, and . . . puddlers purchasing for themselves sealskin waistcoats'[35] were frowned upon in a manner reminiscent of eighteenth-century outcries against 'luxury' and 'extravagance'.

However, this view of the 1870s as a difficult transitional period for the working class needs some qualification. Average real wages had been rising perceptibly since the fifties, so the 1870s did not initiate a rise in real wages, indeed between 1876 and 1882 growth was not sustained. But as Prof. Hobsbawm has pointed out, it is necessary to distinguish the way in which gains were made: by money wages moving ahead of prices, as happened up to and including the 1870s, or by falling prices, as was largely the case during the 1880s and 1890s (see Fig. III). He has suggested that when gains came through rising money wages, they were limited to that section of the work-force which, by virtue of its scarcity and bargaining power embodied in trade union organisation, was able to maintain or increase its money wage. Only when rising real wages came in response to falling prices did all sections of the work-force benefit, during the 1880s and 1890s.[36] This suggests that the unskilled on low incomes, whose consumption patterns were most likely to be rigid and traditional, made no real gains in purchasing power until the 1880s. If they then experienced difficulty in coming to terms with a significant

Figure III: *Money Wages and Real Wages in Britain, 1850-1913*

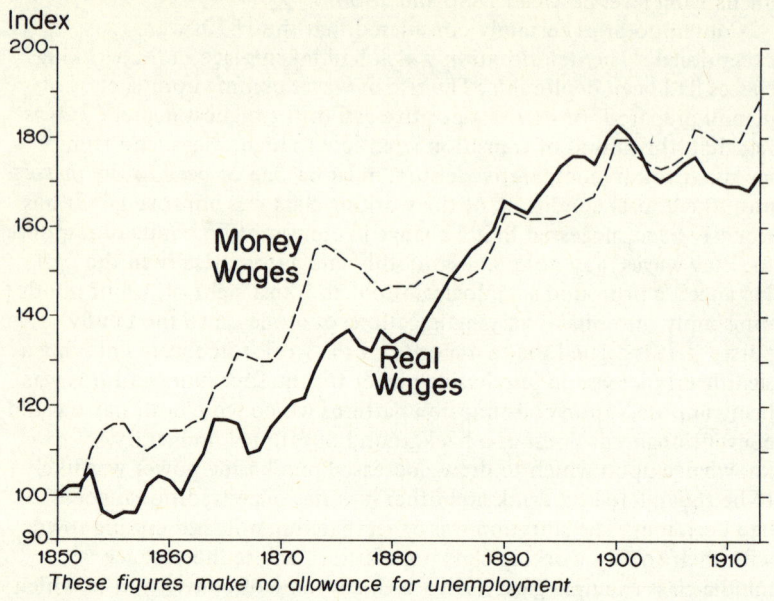

Source: The G.H. Wood series as extended by W.T. Layton and G. Crowther, *An Introduction to the Study of Prices,* 3rd edn., 1938, pp.274-5.

increase in purchasing power for the first time, this was not exhibited by a rise in drink consumption per head. Conversely skilled artisans did experience increasing purchasing power during the seventies, but if they were mainly responsible for the increase, it could not be put down to the difficulties of coming to terms for the first time with the budgetary implications of increased purchasing power, as they had been enjoying rising real wages from the fifties onwards. Some observers did point to the skilled worker as being mainly responsible for the increase in drink consumption during the 1870s. A witness before the *Select Committee on Habitual Drunkards* (1872) explained: 'In Lancashire, which is the highest paid county in the Kingdom, drinking exists to this terrible excess, because a workman can afford to lose one or two days a week, and can yet make a great deal more money than ordinary labourers.'[37] 'Saint Monday' appears to have been a custom which had effectively withstood the more demanding work discipline of an industrial society, at least for skilled artisans.[38]

The second qualification comes in regard to the availability of a wider range of consumer goods on which the rising money wages of the 1870s could be spent. Middle-class contemporaries assumed that these existed, but this is by no means certain. Diet was still largely determined by the state of British agriculture as large-scale imports of cheap foodstuffs had not yet arrived. Improvements in housing conditions for the rapidly growing urban population depended on more than rising wages; it was a question of regulating and improving the whole urban environment and therefore beyond the scope of the individual, however wealthy. As far as consumer durables such as clothing were concerned, these were still being produced by pre-industrial techniques for the middle-class market, and were in a price range beyond the reach of working-class pockets. The inadequacy of existing retailing facilities and methods, with a plethora of small retail establishments in working-class areas, working on low turnovers and high profit margins, was a legitimate grievance. It meant that those who bought in small quantities paid high prices.[39] The only consumer industry which had so far revolutionised its production and distribution methods to take advantage of the growing urban market of cash-paying customers was the brewing industry.[40]

So it is likely that the peak of drink consumption in the 1870s was a response to a situation in which purchasing power had temporarily outstripped the supply of consumer goods available, once basic needs had been satisfied. There was a limit to which people would wish to eat larger quantities of a restricted and boring diet; drink and increased leisure were preferable. This would of course hold true only for those whose income had risen to such an extent that there was surplus purchasing power available once basic needs had been satisfied. This suggests (as do the wage data) that it was the relatively skilled, higher-income wage-earner who pushed up the level of drink consumption in these years. For the unskilled, while they may have been drawn more fully into the economy and enjoyed slightly higher wages, the satisfaction of minimum needs would probably not have left any surplus purchasing power.[41]

The eventual availability of a wider range of consumer goods needs to be viewed in relation to the level of drink consumption after the boom of the 1870s. The initial emergence of a 'mass market' has usually been located in the 1880s with a noticeable change in consumption habits becoming evident.[42] The volume of imported foodstuffs, grain, meat, bacon, dairy products and fruit widened the degree of consumer choice, as did the emergence of a 'delayed industrial revolution'[43] in many consumer goods industries. Cheap mass-produced consumer durables such as boots, shoes and clothing, and food-processing industries such as jam-making grew rapidly. These goods heralded a revolution in retail and distribution techniques with the emergence of multiple retailers working on high turnover and low profit margins per sale. Such developments led to a rapid fall in the price of consumer goods, beginning in the late 1870s but becoming more widespread in the 1880s and 1890s.

The timing of these developments seems to have been determined in the main by changes in supply rather than demand. There was certainly a growth in size of concentrated urban markets, but after reaching a peak in 1874, money wages fell away to 1879 and then showed little change until 1888. But changes on the supply side, the harvest of exported capital, railway networks into the interior of newly settled regions, free trade and improved steamships appear to have been more important. Improved retailing and distribution methods were applied extensively to imported foodstuffs. Indeed only with the use of new methods of handling could perishable imports such as meat and dairy produce be marketed at all. The link between mass-produced consumer durables and new retailing techniques was also close.[44] It was the reduction in prices resulting from these changes which pushed up real wages and created the necessary demand, while money wages were stagnating. This argument for the primacy of supply factors in determining the emergence of a mass market is strengthened by evidence which suggests that some of the new imported commodities such as tinned meat and bananas had to overcome antipathy to them, and generate demand by vigorous sales drives.[45] Furthermore, new methods of production led to the production of goods in anticipation of demand rather than in response to orders, as had previously been the case.[46] So there is little to suggest that expenditure on drink in the 1870s in any way inhibited or delayed these new developments by reducing the level of effective demand for them.

When these wider developments are seen in relation to the pattern of drink consumption shown in Fig. I, two features are evident. Firstly, from the 1880s onwards the range of commodities within reach of the working class was widening considerably, both in variety and in price. Drink, on the other hand, remained unchanged in price, so it was becoming proportionally more expensive relative to an increasingly wide range of alternative consumer goods. Secondly, drink consumption per head rose when an increase in real wages came in response to rising money wages, as occurred in the mid-1870s, 1900, and to a minor extent around 1890 and 1910. But when real wages rose as a result of falling prices between 1880 and 1895, the level of drink consumption stagnated.

In the conditions holding between 1870 and 1876, the price relationship between drink and the limited range of alternative consumer goods available remained substantially unchanged or perhaps moved marginally in favour of drink. Furthermore, the way in which rising purchasing power was achieved, through rising money wages, meant that it first passed through the hands of the main drink consumer within the family before reaching the housewife who was responsible for household purchases. It is therefore probable that some of the increase was spent on drink before reaching the housewife.[47] To the extent that this happened, the purchasing power of the family as a whole was not effectively increased.

In the conditions holding between 1880 and 1895, where rising real wages came largely in response to falling prices, the price relationship between alternative commodities was disturbed. Because of falling food prices, drink was becoming relatively more expensive than it had been previously. This acted as an incentive not to increase expenditure on drink, but to turn instead to the widening range of consumer goods. The effect would tend to be strengthened because increased purchasing power was felt first by the housewife through falling prices allowing her to buy more with her fixed money budget. It was then probably more likely to be effectively utilised than if it had come in the first instance to the main wage-earner and drinker in the family. So between 1880 and 1895 there was a powerful cash incentive to change traditional consumption habits in a way that would maximise the benefits of falling prices in generating an improved standard of living.[48]

There is still the problem of explaining why the levels of drink consumption fell from the peak in 1875-6 to a lower level in the early 1880s before stagnating, rather than simply remaining at the peak level. The temporary halt to the rise in real wages, 1876-82, combined with the fact that retail prices were beginning to fall rapidly (30 per cent between 1877 and 1887), suggests that this was the crucial period in which consumption patterns began to be modified. Cheaper foodstuffs were preferred to drink. When real wages resumed their upward path from 1882 onwards the static level of drink consumption was representative of its changing place in an improving working-class diet. Drink was not alone in this: bread and potato consumption per head also ceased to rise from the early 1880s. The peak in drink consumption around 1900 can be seen as a partial return to conditions holding during the 1870s. A rise in the price of consumer goods from their low point in the 1890s slowed down the rise in real wages and substantial gains were once more being made only by those capable of pushing up their money wages ahead of rising prices. Therefore the price differential between drink and alternative consumer goods was again being narrowed. But the peak in 1900 did not reach the levels of 1876. This suggests that some at least of the *wider* range of alternatives now available, while becoming more expensive relative to drink had become a sufficiently well-established part of working-class consumption patterns to be retained even at higher prices. After 1900 with a stagnation in the level of real wages, the decline in the consumption of drink can be seen as an attempt to safeguard and maintain new consumption habits in which drink now played a lesser role than previously.

The decline was temporarily reversed in the years 1910-14, when money wages rose. Beveridge had warned in 1909 that 'the decrease in the consumption of alcohol in the last ten years has been great enough to justify a hope of permanent improvement, but the hope may be rudely shattered at the next period of general prosperity.'[49] But the significant feature was that drink consumption was still at significantly lower levels than those experienced from 1870 onwards and absorbed a much smaller proportion of total purchasing power than previously.

Table I: *UK Expenditure on Tobacco as a Proportion of Total Consumer Expenditure**

Figures in annual averages per decade

Year	%
1870-9	1.46
1880-9	1.59
1890-9	1.61
1900-9	1.79
1910-14	2.00

* Total consumer expenditure on goods and services at current prices.

Sources: Total consumer expenditure, Jefferys and Walters, op. cit. Expenditure on tobacco, Prest, op. cit., pp.89-91.

Cigarettes were among the most conspicuous of the widening range of commodities which were successfully competing with drink for a larger slice of working-class purchasing power. Total expenditure on tobacco rose from £13.5 million in 1870 to £42 million in 1914. These aggregate figures, however, conceal the dramatic rise in the popularity of cigarettes, particularly after the turn of the century. Expenditure on cigarettes in 1900 was £4.8 million, amounting to about one-fifth of all spending on tobacco; this rose to £23.3 million in 1914, well over half total tobacco expenditure.[50] In spite of this rise the proportion of earnings devoted to tobacco was much smaller than in the case of drink, as Table I indicates. Many contemporaries felt that expenditure on tobacco, like drink, was economically damaging. In contrast to drink, however, there was a gradual but sustained increase in the proportion of income spent on tobacco between 1870 and 1914. This proportion did not fluctuate markedly from year to year; for example, there was no increase during the boom of the seventies, nor any subsequent falling away. Thus tobacco consumption does not appear to have been susceptible to the same kind of factors as those influencing the changing level of drink consumption.

Conclusion

In conclusion, expenditure on drink did affect working-class living standards, by depressing the level of nutrition enjoyed, and being largely responsible for 'the disproportion shown . . . between average earnings and results in the comforts of home'.[51] Furthermore, the high level of taxation on drink meant that the tax burden imposed on the working class was, relative to income, higher than for any other section of society. This was defended on the grounds that these taxes were 'self-imposed' and could therefore be avoided if drink was not purchased. Samuel Smiles regarded this as a positive incentive to stop drinking.[52] But the extent to which drink inhibited rising living standards declined from the 1870s onwards. Even the peak levels during the 1870s need to be seen in relation to the scarcity of alternative consumer goods once basic needs had been satisfied, and the possibility that the more affluent sections of the work-force were mainly responsible for the increase. This group were least likely to be near the poverty line and pushed below it owing to increased drink consumption.

During the 1880s and 1890s the retarding effect of drink expenditure was lessened. While Fig. II shows expenditure remaining between 12 and 13 per cent, the remaining 87 per cent of purchasing power was buying more in real terms as prices fell. The widening range of consumer goods, through their reduced price, generated rising real wages in a way that was not susceptible to erosion by increased expenditure on drink. In this way the foundations for the age of 'high mass consumption' were firmly established. However, while the growth in consumer demand was not positively retarded by rising drink expenditure, neither was it positively assisted by an absolute reduction in this expenditure until after 1900. This suggests that while levels of drink consumption were partially determined by relative price changes of competing commodities, there was also a significant degree of autonomous consumption. This can be regarded as the manifestation of a deep-rooted complex of social and cultural patterns of which drinking was an integral part, and which only slowly responded to economic forces.

The non-economic determinants of the level of drink consumption — the spread of temperance sentiment, the increasing provision of alternative leisure pursuits, the extension of education, and so on[53] — frequently quoted to account for the decline, particularly after 1900, have not been mentioned here. This is not out of a belief that they are unimportant, or that the myth of the 'economic man' offers a sufficient explanation. It is rather that these determinants often cannot be quantified, so making it difficult to demonstrate any relationship. They have been advanced on the assumption that they were alternatives to drink, competing with it for available finance and time. But this assumption of competing alternatives also forms the basis of the explanation offered above. So any explanation of the changing levels of drink consumption in terms of non-economic factors should complement rather than compete with the analysis offered here. But their effects will be assessible only as a result of detailed local studies which examine the role of drink in the diet and recreational activities of the working class.

Temperance reformers and other middle-class critics of the working class in Victorian Britain had a valid case when they pointed to drink as an important threat to the material well-being of the working man. But they pursued their inquiries no further and failed to ask why men drank. The voice of the authentic working man was rarely if every heard on the subject. It was left to socialists to point out that much drinking was a response to a squalid environment rather than a cause of it, thus discrediting temperance reform as the universal panacea for all social ills. If the ameliorative and recreational roles of drink are considered, the case against drink in the nineteenth century is by no means overwhelming. Without easy recourse to 'the quickest road out of Manchester' the pressure for change from below might have come sooner and more insistently than in fact it did in Victorian Britain.

Notes

1. I am grateful to Dr. Brian Harrison and Dr. Lucy Brown who read an earlier draft of this article and made helpful comments.
2. B.S. Rowntree, *Poverty: A Study of Town Life*, 4th edn., 1902, p.140.
3. D.J. Oddy, 'Working-Class Diets in Late Nineteenth-Century Britain', *Economic History Review*, 2nd ser. XXIII (1970) p.322.
4. See for example S.G. Checkland, *The Rise of Industrial Society in England 1815-1885*, Oxford, 1964, p.234; G.M. Trevelyan, *Illustrated English History: The Nineteenth Century*, Penguin edn., 1964, p.206; George J. Barnsby, 'The Standard of Living in the Black Country during the Nineteenth Century', *Econ. Hist. Rev.*, 2nd ser. XXIV (1971), pp.231-2.
5. The statistical evidence available indicates the 1870s as the peak period of beer and spirits consumption, but the statistics for the early part of the century are weak due to the amount of spirits smuggling and illicit distillation and home brewing. Therefore there may have been higher *per capita* peaks in the 1820s and 1830s. I am indebted to Dr. Brian Harrison for this point.
6. G.B. Wilson, *Alcohol and the Nation*, 1940, pp.7-14, 55-60.
7. ibid., p.9.
8. Brian Harrison, 'Drink and Sobriety in England 1815-1872: A Critical Bibliography', *International Review of Social History*, XII (1967), pp.208-9.
9. Joseph Rowntree and Arthur Sherwell, *The Temperance Problem and Social Reform,* 8th edn., 1900, p.84.
10. ibid., pp.5-6.
11. Harrison, op.cit., p.209. Adult membership of the two largest teetotal societies, The Independent Order of Rechabites, and the Sons of Temperance, rose from 23,109 in 1870 to 356,457 in 1910. But in addition to this there were many small teetotal societies often affiliated to churches, and many abstainers were probably not formally linked to any society.
12. A.R. Prest, *Consumers' Expenditure in the United Kingdom 1900-1919*,

Cambridge, 1954, pp.76-80. Duties on spirits were increased in 1909, causing a rise and a temporary reduction in consumption levels.
13. Wilson, op.cit., p.197.
14. op.cit., p.289.
15. See below, p.122.
16. Charles Booth, *Life and Labour of the People in London,* final vol. (AMS Press reprint of 1902-4 edn.), p.70; G.R. Sims, letter in *Daily News,* 24 November 1883; B.S. Rowntree, op.cit., p.143; John Burnett, *Plenty and Want: A Social History of Diet in England from 1915 to the Present Day,* Pelican edn., 1968, p.199.
17. Leone Levi, *Wages and Earnings of the Working Classes,* 1885, p.69.
18. John Yudkin, 'History and the Nutritionist', in T.C. Barker, J.C. McKenzie, J. Yudkin (eds.), *Our Changing Fare: Two Hundred Years of British Food Habits,* 1966, p.157.
19. J.C. Drummond and Anne Wilbraham, *The Englishman's Food,* revised edn., 1958, pp.357, 388-9; cf. Burnett, op.cit., p.142; Barker *et al.,* op.cit., p.27.
20. Brian Harrison, op.cit., p.211. The use of alcohol as a medicine in London hospitals declined markedly from the early 1870s onwards; see Sir Victor Horsley and Mary D. Sturge, *Alcohol and the Human Body,* 5th edn., 1915, pp.4-5.
21. J.H. Bunker, 'The Nutritive Value of Yeast, Beer, Wines and Spirits', *Chemistry and Industry,* 19 April 1947, pp.203-5; cf. Sir Stanley Davidson and R. Passmore, *Human Nutrition and Dietetics,* 3rd edn., reprint 1967, Ch.7.
22. Charles Booth, *Labour and Life of the People,* 1, 3rd edn., 1891, p.135.
23. See below, pp.128-9.
24. W.A. MacKenzie, 'Changes in the Standard of Living in the United Kingdom 1860-1914', *Economica,* no.3 (1921).
25. ibid., pp.223-5.
26. Method of calculating calorific value of beer as suggested by H.J. Bunker, op.cit., p.203, assuming an average specific gravity of $1055°$.
27. See above, p.120.
28. Regional variations in the consumption of spirits make the inclusion of spirits in the example rather difficult. But on the assumption that 30 per cent of all working-class drink expenditure went on spirits and the rest on beer (see p.117, the resultant reduction in calorific intake would rise slightly to 18.3 per cent. A further assumption made was that all alcohol consumed was effectively utilised in the body to provide energy. This is likely to have been true only under favourable circumstances; see Bunker, op.cit., p.204; Davidson and Passmore, op.cit., pp.113-14.
29. Booth, *Labour and Life,* 1, pp.146-8; Rowntree, op.cit., p.142.
30. *Select Committee on Habitual Drunkards...* Parl. Papers 1872, IX, p.3, QQ. 1729-31; *S.C. House of Lords on the Prevalence of Habits of Intemperance...* P.P. 1877, XI, QQ. 647, 720-23, 9729-30.
31. A.D. Webb, 'The Consumption of Alcoholic Liquors in the United Kingdom', *Journal Royal Statistical Society,* LXXVI (1912-13), p.216; D.S. Thomas, *Social Aspects of the Business Cycle,* New York, 1927, Ch.7.
32. Samuel Smith, President of Liverpool Chamber of Commerce, quoted in *27th Annual Report of the United Kingdom Alliance* (1879), p.45; Goldwin Smith, 'The Labour Movement', *Contemporary Review,* XXI (Jan. 1873), p.250; Anon., 'The Proletariat on a False Scent', *Quarterly Review,* CXXIII, no. 263 (Jan. 1872), p.279.
33. S.G. Checkland, op.cit., p.233.
34. ibid. pp.232-3; cf. S. Pollard, *A History of Labour in Sheffield,* Liverpool, 1959, p.23.
35. Levi, op.cit., p.36.

36. E.J. Hobsbawm, *Industry and Empire*, Pelican edn., 1969, p.162; cf. his *Labouring Men*, 1968 edn., pp.293-4; R.S. Tucker, 'Real Wages of Artisans in London, 1729-1935', *Journal of American Statistical Society*, XXXI (1936), p.84. In the absence of more detailed information on wages and employment during the boom of the early 1870s it is impossible to gauge to what extent the level of unemployment among the unskilled fell, or if their money wages moved up appreciably.
37. op.cit., Q. 707.
38. ibid. Q. 706; cf. [Thomas Wright], *Some Habits and Customs of the Working Classes by a Journeyman Engineer*, 1867, for an indication of the importance of drink in the working life and recreational activities of skilled artisans. See especially p.125, for a description of 'Saint Mondayites'.
39. 'The Proletariat on a False Scent', loc. cit., pp.286-90.
40. P. Mathias, *Retailing Revolution*, 1967, p.7.
41. This is not of course meant to suggest that the unskilled did not drink, but that they were not in a position to increase their customary level of drink expenditure significantly.
42. Burnett, op.cit., p.132.
43. J.B. Jefferys, *Retail Trading in Britain 1850-1950*, Cambridge, 1954, p.8; cf. Charles Wilson, 'Economy and Society in Late Victorian Britain', *Econ. Hist. Rev.*, 2nd ser. XVIII (1965), p.189, who coined the phrase 'revolution of the domestic economy'.
44. ibid., p.190.
45. Betty McNamee, 'Trends in Meat Consumption', p.81, and Angeliki Torode, 'Trends in Fruit Consumption', p.126, both in Barker *et al.*, op.cit.; cf. Pollard, op.cit., p.107.
46. Jefferys, op.cit., p.8.
47. Booth, *Labour and Life*, 1, p.139; idem, *Life and Labour*, final vol., p.70; Checkland, op.cit., p.235.
48. 'Probably the keenness of price competition would not have been expressed so forcibly, and probably the habits of buying new products not acquired so rapidly, had the gain in money wages been slow and steady, without setbacks or lulls . . . Income conditions for the masses, which both increased their range of purchasing and sharpened their appreciation of lower prices, were to their advantage.' – Mathias, op.cit., pp.13-14.
49. *Employment: A Problem of Industry*, 1930 edn., p.46.
50. Prest, op.cit., pp.89-91.
51. Booth, *Life and Labour*, 2nd ser., V, p.334.
52. Levi, op.cit., p.65. Samuel Smiles, *Self-Help*, 1878 edn., p.292; cf. 'The Proletariat on a False Scent', loc. cit., pp.269-70.
53. Wilson, op.cit., Ch. 22, for a comprehensive list of factors thought to affect the level of drink consumption.

11 REGIONAL VARIATIONS IN FOOD HABITS

D.E. ALLEN

Introduction

Quantitative information on diet in the past is hard to come by and tends to be fragmentary at best. Understandably, therefore, historians have learned to be thankful for what they have and hardly see fit to ask awkward questions about such luxury aspects as geographical representativeness. It is not the custom of historians, in any case, to sieve their data in spatial terms. Their traditional raw material is very seldom so copious and complete that it lends itself to such analysis, and even when this does prove possible the very sparsity of comparable examples robs the findings of much meaning. In so far as there is historical work in regional terms at all at present, this consists of the building up of an almost wholly qualitative picture out of a multiplicity of local detail — as opposed to a quantitative segmentation of national data. The region of the historian is still essentially the parish or market town or individual county writ large: it is not yet a level of analysis that exists in its own right. There is no established practice of breaking down the national picture and checking, much less measuring, the degree to which the pictures of the several parts bear out the picture of the whole. Yet for forty years now, since Crawford and Broadley published their pioneer survey of *The People's Food*,[1] quantitative data of a novel and rather special type have been accumulating in this very field of tastes and eating habits that increasingly make possible generalisations at an infra-national level. Forty years back from the present, of course, scarcely ranks as what historians are accustomed to thinking of as 'history'. But before much longer the data will have gathered sufficient dust and venerability to be thought worthy of consideration, and in anticipation of that time it may be useful to provide some foretaste of what those researchers of the future may expect to find.

The data in question come from sample surveys. This method has been in use for the study of British society since as far back as 1912; it began to catch on in the 1920s but, for complex historical reasons, till only very recently its application has been predominantly commercial. This latter fact has been partly responsible for a general academic neglect of the results. Just because a survey has been carried out under commercial conditions, it has been tempting to assume that corners must have been cut and that the methodology must be untrustworthy. The necessarily streamlined character of such work and the traditional reliance of market researchers on quota samples, as opposed to the random samples insisted on by purists, have further contributed to this suspicion. Yet much commercial survey work continues to be fact-gathering of the simplest kind, aimed at establishing nothing more ambitious than the proportion of different segments of the population owning or using particular consumer products. There are, of course, pitfalls for the careless or inexperienced even in this. But just because of its very simplicity this work has the great asset that many of its findings are all the time being unwittingly replicated. It is thus possible to check the general degree of accuracy of surveys of this kind — and it is fair to say that from any such scrutiny they tend to emerge reasonably unscathed. As it is these surveys that yield by far the greatest part of the data on regional food preferences and habits, there would thus seem ample justification for drawing on their results. At the same time it goes without saying that this must be done with care; for though alluringly quantitative this is relatively 'soft' data compared with what economists are accustomed to, the occasional freak figure is a built-in hazard of the sampling method and there is always the chance as well that the survey has emerged from a chronically inaccurate stable.

A far greater cause of neglect, however, is the general inaccessibility of the results of commercial surveys to the non-commercial world. The problem is not just that so much is carried out for private clients and thus has to be kept confidential — or else is made available at a more or less prohibitive price. Far more in fact is published than is popularly supposed. The deeper problem is that this publication is so often limited and obscure in the extreme, confined to the release of a mere handful of copies to those lucky enough to have spotted the relevant small paragraph in that particular week's trade press. If only this difficulty can be surmounted, an almost bewilderingly rich and varied harvest is assured. Government data, most notably the National Food Survey (analysed regionally since 1955), can be drawn on extensively to supplement this.

By a piece of luck, the subdivision of the country employed in most of these surveys has long been basically the same, namely varying combinations of the Registrar General's Standard Regions. For geographical purposes, therefore, a high degree of comparability between surveys has been unintentionally achieved. It is thus possible to extract the regional data from each one and gradually build up a composite picture, after the manner of aerial photographers with their mosaics of overlays. Just as in aerial photography, numerous patterns that are invisible on the ground at once spring to sight when recourse is had to this method. Only by means of the sample survey is it possible to detect the small proportional discrepancies between one part of the country and another of which most regional difference in Britain is nowadays made up. Only rarely are the contrasts sufficiently large and definite to present themselves to the eye unaided. And even more rarely is the difference of an absolute order of magnitude rather than merely relative. To accumulate sufficient data to yield a reasonably detailed picture, it is necessary to draw on surveys extending over a span of several years. Even with the great volume of survey work now proceeding the amount of published material is still much too slight to allow one to think in terms of adequate 'snapshots' at appreciably more frequent intervals. Although the annual character of the National Food Survey and the regular surveys of expenditure on branded food products put out by IPC Magazines Ltd. might appear to belie this, the scope of these is inevitably very restricted and the picture they are capable of providing, even jointly, is far too insubstantial to be at all comparable.

The one major study on these lines that has so far been published[2] ranged over a whole decade, 1955-65, for the greater part of the survey data on which it was based – and even then sizeable gaps in information remained. So broad a time-span does have the advantage of enabling many changes that are no more than transient (or mere freaks of sampling) to be identified and discounted. On the other hand it is obviously open to the danger of presenting a misleadingly static picture. The speed of change today is such that many regional differences, however long-enduring in the past, may now be crumbling away inside so brief a space as ten years. And ten further years have elapsed, what is more, since the period of the study in question. Nevertheless, it is hard to believe that the broader patterns it disclosed have been significantly modified in recent years. The closer one looks, the more these broader patterns appear suggestive of deep-seated continuities, some of which have surely held good even for many centuries. Despite the apparently dated nature of the study, therefore, it seems well worth while bringing the more salient of these to the notice of nutritionists and historians.

North versus South

The broadest of these patterns is the simple dichotomy between North and South. A lot of alleged North/South differences are of course spurious, based on a fallacious conception of 'the North'. The North/South dichotomy referred to here is a demonstrable gradation of difference as one moves up through the country from one end to the other – that is to say, the far South of England represents one pole and Scotland the other. There are several possible causes of this pattern. One, clearly, is climate: as one travels northwards it becomes progressively colder. This naturally finds its most marked and wide-ranging reflection in the fields of clothing and bedding, but it also has some effect on food: hotter seasons in the South tend to drive out soup, ordain more ice-cream and salads, and mean more home-grown fruit. However, other major determinants such as social class complicate the picture. The North is more preponderantly working-class, some two-fifths of its population being classified as semi-skilled or unskilled as against about a third who belong to the professional and managerial classes — proportions which in the South are neatly reversed. The South, in other words, is socially more heterogeneous — and this, too, can be demonstrated statistically. The South's greater openness to innovation, its greater receptivity to new ideas, is possibly a direct result of this — though it does of course happen to possess the country's capital and is fortunate to be the end situated closest to the Continent.

The narrower range of jobs in the North (which is tied up with the concentration there of the heavier industries) also serves to increase the uniformity of tastes and interests on either side of what tends to be a more hard-and-fast social iron curtain. This in turn is tied up with a difference in mobility. On the whole people in the North are much more likely to have grown up with one another. The family, as an institution, thrives more in the North and stretches further. There is a greater tendency there for people to live among relations and long-established family friends. A survey on weddings has shown that people in the North continue to be less likely to marry a comparative stranger than people in the South. All of this leads to greater 'mateyness': to a more engulfing sense of community, to less reserve in social relations but at the same time less willingness to experiment, less of a welcome for the new-fangled.

Underlying this is a difference in the personality type prevailing. For reasons we do not really understand Northerners (and here we must include Midlanders as well) tend to be harsher and more puritanical. The North favours stiffer brushes, coarser suitings, harsher surfaces. Northerners tend to be chewers of sweets, Southerners suckers. Psychologists who have conducted attitude studies in different regional centres have also found that Northerners tend to react in more black-and-white terms, have generally more pronounced and positive opinions. This may reflect their puritanism; alternatively, it may be a reflection of the lower threshold for nuances typical of the less sophisticated. For Northerners (it is no secret) are more blunt and straightforward — in their tastes no less than in their manner. They demand stronger beer, because they drink beer for what it does to them rather than to ponder the subtleties of flavour. In the same way, when they buy a product such as Gorgonzola, they are known to go for a minimum mould on it. The prefer things that make immediate sense: plain, homely fare, without suspicious-sounding ingredients, fussy additions or fancy names. One of the first surveys I was ever involved in myself was on meat and fish pastes. It was fascinating to see how the Northerners tended to turn up their noses at all the more esoteric combinations — chicken-and-ham, sardine-and-anchovy — and plumped, almost infallibly, for the 'no-nonsense', tried-and-trusted flavours: ham, salmon, beef — or even, plainly and simply, 'meat'. The Northerner would prefer to feel that what he eats does him good: he looks for nourishment value in what would scarcely occur to the average Southerner as more than a tasty variety. Soup for the Northerner is very much a food, so (apart from nationally-shared tastes like tomato) he keeps to safe, familiar flavours — once again — like chicken, kidney and celery. Any soft drink that can be convincingly claimed to have health-giving properties will sell best in the North, the mere refreshers best in the South. The North, presumably for this reason, is the major market for vitamin pills. The liking for more 'body' in food and drink may explain why Northern tastes also tend to run to darker colours. This is known in products as varied as beer, boiled sweets, icing sugar and (at any rate formerly) rum. The belief that the deeper the colour of the yolk, the better the egg also finds more Northern subscribers.

The Northerner is also less keen on variety. Indeed, there is a detectable monolithic tendency running through many areas of Northern behaviour. The fewer meals — with more eaten per sitting, for example — are nicely paralleled by tastes at the cinema: back in the days when there was still ample scope for local variation, the North specialised in single-feature programmes and the films screened there more often ran full-length; the South, in its typically more restless fashion, demanded more variety for its money and had less objection to cutting.

'Variety is the spice of life' can only be a Southerner's saying, in fact. The South is the land of mixtures, of experimental mingling — jelly and blancmange together as a single dish, for example — and of subtler flavours: saltier bacon, more pungent types of cheese, more bitter marmalade, dry wines, even spinach. All in all, the South is more *specialised:* life there has evolved more distinctions, sprouted more branches and twigs. It is also more 'personalised': bacon sold in ready-cut strips, rarely if ever sliced on the counter from a communal roll; butter in separately wrapped slabs, rather than (as formerly so often in the North) chunks 'off the lump'. It prefers things to be distinctive, to provide means of standing apart from the generalised, anonymous mass. It is, in short, more middle-class.

The North's more rigid texture, its greater homogeneity, the fact that it tends to be more all-of-a-piece, means that it cannot absorb novelty on the scale, or at the speed, of the South — even supposing that it wanted to. Its greater resistance to the more deep-rooted types of innovation, however, means that, paradoxically, it is mainly the relatively shallow things, the 'froth', the inessentials of varying degrees of triviality, which percolate most easily through the social filters and constitute the most obviously visible movement northwards. A good deal of this consists of luxury, or at any rate reasonably sophisticated products which are natural candidates for adoption as status symbols — and which, because of the smaller size of the 'smart' sets in the North, have less success in penetrating. Indeed, just by studying what the North rejects, or the relative speed at which it accepts, we can equip ourselves with remarkably faithful instruments for gauging the ups and downs of its prejudices at different periods. Old fashions that linger on in the North and take an unconscionably long time a-dying may be presumed *prima facie* to betray, by this very fact, a special emotional or functional value in the regional context over and above their original innocent expression. Equally, for a new fashion to start in the North and only later spread southwards is so contrary to the standard pattern as to suggest some extra dimension of super-utility or symbolism. There are just two properly documented examples of this rare phenomenon that I have been able to track down: the 1960s 'Beatlemania' and in the eighteenth century the eating of potatoes.

Highland versus Lowland

Another, almost equally broad pattern exists in a kind of transverse relationship to the more conspicuous North/South one. This is the dichotomy between the Highland Zone of the North and West and the Lowland Zone of the South and East, reflecting the sharp natural cleavage slantwise across Great Britain between the older and the younger rocks, between predominantly acid and predominantly neutral or calcareous soils, between soft water and hard water, between the bare, bleak up-country — essentially a land of hill-grazings — and the lush water-meadows and rolling cornfields. Throughout history this has been the true major dichotomy as far as geography is concerned. In terms of crops it has meant an age-old division into the oat-lands of the North and West and the barley- and wheat-lands of the South and East. Soil and climate have remained inexorable, with only relatively brief and relatively minor oscillations, for thousands of years, ordaining this basic pattern. And although the dichotomy in practices and tastes that this division has given rise to has been substantially eroded down the years, it still stubbornly asserts itself to an extent that is commonly overlooked.

One of the best examples of this is the failure of beer, that beverage of the barley zone, to swamp altogether the pastoralists' allegiance to milk. Pastoral peoples all the world over reckon status in terms of the size of herds: cattle are killed for meat as sparingly as possible and milk in consequence, in blander climates, tends to be in perpetual surplus. The Welsh, a pastoral people *par excellence,* traditionally built a lot of their cooking around milk and cheese as a result. Even today this is a region with an exceptionally high consumption of milk puddings (producing a strong demand in consequence for rice). In the West Country, for the same reason, we find a prolific, even prodigal use of cream (they even pour it over vegetables there). Professor W.G. Hoskins tells me that the commercial production of cream can be traced back to the thirteenth century in Devon. I understand, too, that pilchards and cream is an authentic Cornish dish. But cooking was never capable of absorbing the whole of the surplus: the rest simply had to be drunk — and on such a scale that there can have been room for very little else. There is a nice piece of evidence, indeed, that to the Welsh, at least, beer and spirits were essentially alien. In 1277, when their leader, Llywellyn ap Gruffydd, went up to London to pay homage to the English King (Edward I), his considerable retinue of Welshmen startled their hosts at Islington by spurning the London beer — and demanding milk instead. Today, both Wales and the West Country consistently exhibit a well above-average consumption of liquid milk.

In the same way, just as oven-baked bread has now spread throughout Britain more or less universally, ousting the thin quarter-circles or 'farls', made without yeast, that once prevailed in the West, the old oat culture still dictates the porridge of the Scots (and, to a lesser extent, of the Lancastrians) as well as Scotland's distinctive biscuit confectionery. The Scots' predilection for soups and marked liking for pulses, equally, spring from the ancient stewing/steaming/simmering tradition of the permanent pot on the hearth — a tradition that still lies behind cooking methods throughout the North and West. Pressure-cookers, for example, are much more popular there; special types of potato are favoured because of their capacity to boil without first breaking up; and, compared with the Midlands and South, vegetables are more often steamed and more often shredded before being tossed into pans. In 1797 Sir Frederick Eden pointed to the better diet enjoyed by labourers in the North of England due to the great variety of cheap and savoury soups; their Southern counterparts, by contrast, were never in the habit of boiling meat for stock. Today, still, we find the Northerner preferring to boil or stew where the Southerner roasts or grills: the cooking-pot, in other words, still obstinately holding out against the advance of the oven.

The suggestion has been made by a leading authority on folk life, Professor Estyn Evans,[3] that the cooking-pot on the hearth is a direct descendant of the Bronze Age cauldrons familiar to archaeologists (comparable, say, with the West Room of the Celtic homestead) and carefully handed down within families. In upland, pastoral Britain, the hearth was the focal centre for the household — not the kitchen table. Tables in that part of the country consequently still tend to be small, preferably folding away; sometimes they are lacking altogether. In compensation, there are large pieces of furniture on the periphery, like the Welsh dresser or the huge sink of Scotland with its double draining-board. The lowland English, by contrast, were prepared to disregard the hearth, centering their existence on 'the board', the place where the bread was taken from the oven and carved, sitting round in a circle facing one another. There are two fundamentally different cultures at work here, with roots that must stretch back many hundreds of years.

Because for pastoral peoples cattle are all-important, tillage tends to be neglected, relegated to small plots adjoining the home. As a result both the Scots and the Welsh have a poorly-developed tradition of eating fresh green vegetables — or spending money on seeds or flowers. Their harsher climate, moreover, inhibited the eating of much fresh fruit as well as the development of the English taste for salads. On the other hand, a history of self-sufficiency in farming must presumably explain their constantly heavy consumption of eggs. It is difficult to understand, however, why they share such a distaste for fish and chips or why — without any baking tradition — they are both now such heavy consumers of bread. Salt is also a pre-eminently Welsh and Scottish partiality. Some must accompany all their eggs, of course, and a good deal must go into their soups and stews; but it may also be significant that butter in the Highland Zone has traditionally been saltier than that produced in Lowland England. My guess is that in a certain degree there is a hang-over from the general salting tradition that, for cattle breeders, played so important a part in life before the days of canning. Only meat that had been salted could be wholly depended upon for soundness: 'butcher's meat', indeed, was formerly a favourite Welsh expression of abuse. This extraordinary reverence for foods that have been preserved, irrespective of their reputability nutritionally, turns up in a big way among the Welsh. To account for this, the hypothesis I offer is that the people of Wales, perhaps from very early religious usage, are the victims of an exaggerated concern with purity, which has given them, *inter alia,* a general abhorrence of carelessly treated food. Tinning and freezing, from this point of view, appear as guarantees of safety — and safety, as far as food is concerned, is for the Welsh the overriding consideration. The quite outstanding prestige of pharmacy in Wales may be attributable to this same deep-seated predisposition.

Oddly, the pattern in Scotland in this respect is entirely different. The Scots positively go out of their way to buy made-up meats, pies, cakes, ice-cream — all manner of processed things. At the same time they have proved exceptionally resistant to frozen foods (they were also the most resistant to chilled and frozen meat between the wars) and are unaccountably choosy when it comes to buying tins: tinned soups, baked beans, spaghetti, sweet puddings, fruit juices are entirely acceptable, but tinned fish, peas, fruit, milk and cream are all, for some mysterious reason, bought in very low quantities. It looks as if

Scots housewives, despite their having to produce more and larger meals a day on average than their English counterparts, have managed to persuade themselves that these new types of convenience foods mostly suffer from defects from which their standbys from the butcher or the baker round the corner can safely be assumed to be free. But how has it come about, in that case, that the Scots trust the produce of their local tradesmen, while the Welsh so vehemently revile them? Is there some sharp distinction between these two peoples in their historical experience of retailing?

In Scotland, for a long time, pigs and all their products appear to have been taboo. The result of this today is that both pork and bacon are eaten to a far lesser extent than in any other part of Britain; beef sausages preponderate in the ratio 4 : 1 (against 1 beef : 2 pork in England and Wales as a whole); and branded cooking fats are substituted almost entirely for lard. Admittedly, beef sausages, with their lower meat content, tend to be considerably cheaper than their pork equivalent and are thereby guaranteed a certain privileged access to the notoriously tight purse of the Scots. This explanation, however, will scarcely take us very far — nor will the lack of a tradition in Scotland of roasting and frying. The natural environment, similarly, offers no easy way out: for it appears to present no real barrier to pig-breeders. In desperation, a fossilised religious prohibition, descended from a fundamentalist over-literal reading of the scriptures, has even been suggested, although it receives no support from authorities on Scottish history. For the present, therefore, there remains a mystery.

Yet to treat Scotland as just a region is facile and misleading. It was of course a quite separate country in the not-very-distant past, with cultural traditions that were all the more distinct for having been derived in part from overseas. Relics of the French link are hard to spot now, though at one time — if the social historians are to be believed — they were widespread and obtrusive. Scottish cooking as a whole is said to have received influences from this direction — and certainly the custom of serving a dessert course, of fruit and sweets, is known to have become well-established in Scotland some time before it made its appearance in England. However, the advent of strict Presbyterianism, round about 1650, doubtless halted everything French in its tracks. Much less well-known (at any rate in England), and evidently a good deal more widespread and lasting in its effects, is the longstanding connection between Scotland and Sweden. In large part because of this Swedish influence the North-East of Scotland is today noticeably distinct, with different traditions and different orientations in business. This area has presumably acted as a funnel for various tastes and habits of manifest Scandinavian affinity which have become diffused through Scotland very widely. Because Scotland belongs climatically in the same Nordic Zone, however, it is difficult to be sure that some at least of these influences did not enter much earlier. The subject is an intriguing one and deserves more detailed study.

Tyneside and the Midlands

This kind of interplay between two cultures, and the particular classes of traits which pass most successfully from one to the other, is naturally of especial interest to the cultural anthropologist. By far the best case of this in Britain is the predictably rich Anglo-Scottish amalgam to be found in the area centred on Tyneside. Superficially, the affinities here tend to be with Scotland rather than with England — and this would seem to be no more than appropriate in view of the fact that the inhabitants of the northern half of Northumberland are entirely Scottish on the evidence of their blood-groups. The types of meat and fish most eaten tend to be those most preferred in Scotland; there is the same great liking for both plain and chocolate biscuits, for root vegetables, for butter beans. And this trend in food is echoed in numerous other aspects of life as well. Then, looking harder, we begin to notice discrepancies. The biscuits include the greatest quantity of cream crackers to which Yorkshire is strongly partial, but very few — like Yorkshire again — of the Scotsman's savoury varieties. The oatmeal bought is at the English level, implying no particular fondness for porridge. As in Yorkshire, too, there is a heavy usage of both flour and cooking fats. Fish cakes, malt bread and canned tomatoes, all favourites south of the Tees, are also much esteemed. Most kinds of green vegetables find their way on to the table on a far wider scale than in Scotland and there is an equally un-Scottish acceptance of pig products, such as bacon, Spam and pork sausages — the last competing here, in a nicely compromising fashion, on level terms with the beef variety so heavily preferred in Scotland. The tastes in drink, likewise, are on the whole English. All in all, it is the more structurally rooted traditions, such as the whole complex of home baking, that turn out to look towards the South, suggesting that of the two, it is the Scottishness, rather, that forms the intrusive pattern.

Yet, as in that other fascinating area of overlap, the Midlands, Tyneside can boast of one or two traits that are wholly peculiar to itself: an astonishing capacity (and, presumably, liking) for tinned peas; a quite exceptional demand for corned beef; and by far the heaviest consumption of brown bread in the country, accounting for some 10 per cent of all bread eaten — compared with only about 5 per cent everywhere else in Britain. Milk and cheese, by contrast, show consumptions lower even than in either Yorkshire or Scotland. Some display of independence, however, is perhaps only to be expected of an area like this, much of which enjoyed substantial political autonomy for no less than five centuries.

The fact that these boundary areas are more than just mosaics of the two dominant cultures that lie on either side and possess in fact a far from negligible distinctiveness of their own is probably the most striking finding to emerge from my study. Indeed, before this I suspect that no one had appreciated how very strongly distinctive is that much-misunderstood region, the Midlands. One of the many odd features of the Midlands is the remarkable sourness of the diet. Sales are poor of most sweet things, such as cakes, fruit, fruit juices, cider, sweet biscuits, sweet pastry and all sweet spreads not even excluding jam. The place of these last is taken partly by meat extracts and partly by cheese-and-pickles (which in some parts are even eaten for breakfast — a meal in the Midlands in many cases quite devoid of jam or marmalade and with an altogether savoury tang to it). The acidity of pickles in the Black Country is said to be twice as high as is standard in London. Strong Cheddar very often accompanies them, eaten in solid chunks. Spending on vinegar is the highest in the country, and yet despite this there is also a great fondness for tomato ketchup and that one solitary Midland contribution to the national diet, Worcester sauce. Even the Midland 'mild' is a noticeably more bitter beer than what passes under this name further south. Midlanders make up for this general deficiency of sugar by using quite ridiculous amounts of it in their tea and coffee. In this they reportedly resemble the Brazilians, who similarly manage to combine a liking for heavily sugared coffee with the drinking of great quantities of sourish beer. Overall, one would guess, the Midlands diet contains less sugar than that of any region in Britain, but this has yet to be demonstrated statistically. In the event of this proving to be the case, it may be worth drawing attention to the fact that three separate sets of medical statistics have indicated a remarkably low rate of coronary heart disease among men in the Black Country towns. As Midland men are notably heavy smokers, some other factor than tobacco evidently needs to be involved to explain this apparent inverse correlation. I suggest that it may be a heavy intake of sugar that in other areas serves to tilt the scales.

There are many other regional patterns that seem historically suggestive. The diet of Lancashire, for instance: so utterly unlike that of Yorkshire, semi-'Celtic' in fact in its addiction to stews and with its relic liking for porridge. In its fondness for bought cakes, as well, Lancashire aligns itself markedly with Scotland. The bun-and-pudding diet of Yorkshire, on the other hand, finds echoes in East Anglia: both stretches of the country notable for big, burly people of predominantly Anglo-Saxon stock. In so far as the present-day distribution of manifestly different physical types points to certain regions having had a sharply different racial history, it is tempting to hypothesize some necessary connection between this naturally massive build and this emphasis on bulk in the diet (though I am not of course suggesting that it is the diet that gives rise to the build). In the West Country I have the impression (and it is no more than an impression) that there is some extra emotiveness attached to fruit. For centuries this has been the cradleland of British orchardry, and there is a wealth of ritual and superstition testifying to some very special strength in this cultural link. Again, I find it easier to suppose some long-enduring, if now vestigial, element of veneration rather than assume a gross cultural discontinuity.

Conclusions

From all that anthropology has been able to tell us about the dynamics of cultural interaction, on the strength of evidence drawn from many parts of the world, we know that cooking and eating habits and the central core of diet are among the more resistant to modification or displacement. It is in the nature of food tastes not to change drastically or rapidly over time. It thus makes more sense to presuppose very considerable continuity and a minimum of switching over. If genetic influences play a part as well, then this viewpoint is immeasurably strengthened.

An alternative way of looking at the matter is to examine the degree of change that has occurred in the British diet, in terms of the numerous standard items covered in the National Food Survey, over the last thirty years — a period of enormous technological progress and unprecedented commercial pressures. The change, it will be found, has been amazingly slight, at any rate as far as the *regional* ratios are concerned. From this fact I infer that the regional differences are unlikely to be haphazard, that in such a key sphere as food indeed they are almost bound to be linked in meaningful clusters of more or less long standing, that even where novelties are introduced these are liable to be fitted into some pre-existing, vacant slot. Cultures, in fact — even mere regional cultures — have enormous resilience: man is a creature of habit, and habits die hard. And unless we have wholesale displacement of populations, it is more probable than not that the distinctiveness of regions will hang together and persist.

The regions are nothing like so distinct today as once they were. With so much mobility, with so much exposure to the uniformity of mass media, a great deal has inevitably been lost. Even so, a great deal also still survives. And if so much diversity can manage to persist in a cultural climate so highly adverse as that of today, the tenaciousness of these several regional cultures must be great indeed. In the absence of these pressures, how much more distinct and impervious to new influences they must have been in the past. In view of so much difference, indeed, I wonder how far it really makes sense to speak and write in terms of *national* aggregates at all in a field such as nutrition. Even more, in trying to carry back a subject like this historically, it seems to me all but obligatory to attempt the reconstruction (so far as the records make this feasible) on a basis that is primarily regional.

Notes

1. Sir William Crawford and H. Broadley, *The People's Food,* London, Heinemann, 1938. Based on a consumer survey by Sales Research Services Ltd.
2. D. Elliston Allen, *British Tastes: An Enquiry into the Likes and Dislikes of the Regional Consumer,* London, Hutchinson, 1968. The data cited in the present paper are taken almost wholly from this work, to which the reader is accordingly referred for fuller details and references to sources.
3. E. Estyn Evans, *Irish Folk Ways,* London, Routledge, 1957.

12 THE CORNER SHOP: THE DEVELOPMENT OF THE GROCERY AND GENERAL PROVISIONS TRADE

JANET BLACKMAN

Albert Cattle built up his grocer's business between the two world wars at two different addresses in Hull, and probably started his apprenticeship in the early years of this century. How big a business it was we do not know; the papers he left were nearly all his speaker's notes as a lay preacher with no accounts of his trade.[1] But his books! He clearly took his trade seriously, took a pride in its many-sidedness, and collected a small reference library of grocer's manuals. There were histories of tea and coffee growing and processing, of cheese-making, etc., guides to the 'goods of the grocer and provision dealer',[2] *Law's Grocer's Manual* running to over a thousand pages,[3] and several large illustrated books on window display, lettering, trade card designs and packaging, some with their samples of coloured crepe paper carefully sewn in, and layouts for complete window displays for the shopkeeper to copy.[4] He also bought in the 1930s many of the New Left Book Club studies. He was clearly an interesting tradesman, full of life and probably of opinions too on a variety of subjects. How typical he was of grocers it is hard to tell, but his collection of books does give us some idea of what a keen grocer expected of himself, the kind of skills he acquired and the aids that were available to him from other practitioners in the trade. In some of the books he has signed his name 'Albert Cattle, MGF'—member of the Grocers' Federation, a federation formed in 1891 by linking together the various local grocers' associations, which had been founded partly in response to the prosecution of grocers under the Adulteration of Food Acts of 1872.[5] Albert Cattle was therefore a member of a trade group which took a pride in its skills, was attempting almost to professionalise them, seeking to establish both standards of trading and some form of collective protection to safeguard their trading position. The frontispiece in *Law's Grocer's Manual* is a picture of a very large jolly man captioned 'a model groceryman, always cheerful! and always busy!!'; that of Aubrey Rees's *The Grocery Trade, its History and Romance* is a photograph of the ornate and dignified Grocers' Hall in London.

This is a study therefore of a particular part of the service sector, which in many ways came to reflect by the latter part of the nineteenth century some of the most important ideas and features of a free trade, urbanised economy. The grocery and provision trade had begun to include a range of businesses from the successfully expanding multiples, co-operative stores, large local grocers with more than one shop down to the corner shop, a general store or a small shop in a converted front room of a house. This range of trade was regarded by many contemporary observers, such as George Dodd writing on the food supply of London in the 1850s,[6] as the hallmark of a free trade economy, offering numerous opportunities to the enterprising man or woman. Their chances of failure and of bankruptcy, in a working-class area for instance dependent for its employment on a particular firm or industry, were rarely mentioned; instead, the development of packaged goods, of retail sales techniques, display and advertising, selective pricing and mark-ups according to class of trade began to pull all types of grocery traders together into a particular style of business management.

'Grocer' probably comes from the same root as the word 'gross', meaning 'in bulk'. The old French word, *grossier* was used to denote one who buys and sells in the gross, a wholesale dealer or merchant. This gives an important clue to the style of trading of the traditional grocer. He has long been regarded primarily as a retailer, but in two important ways he remained until recent times a dealer in bulk. Many retail grocers acted as wholesalers by buying in bulk and then breaking down the consignment for other shops in the area as well as for their own branch shops. Rail carriage may have encouraged this; in the 1860s a Sheffield grocer was providing this service to other grocers in the town.[7] And then secondly, the retail grocer was for a very long time himself a processor and packer, buying his tea, sugar, currants, etc. in large quantities, and making them up into smaller amounts for the customer.

Grocers have also for centuries been associated with foreign produce imported into this country by trading companies. The English (London) Company of Grocers in the Middle Ages was made up of merchants dealing in spices, dried fruit, etc. In the seventeenth century tea, coffee and cocoa were added to their main stocks, and with sugar became the most important items in the grocer's trade. As a result until the middle years of the nineteenth century the specialist grocer drew his customers from the middle and higher income groups.

There was a clear distinction in the food trades between the grocer as a dealer in spices, dried fruit, condiments, tea, etc., and the traders in butter, cheese and bacon, etc. The latter were provision dealers, and within this group there was further specialisation. Just as some grocers were specialist tea dealers, there were provision merchants who were butter factors, or cheesemongers. Tooke in his study of prices printed in 1823 defined 'provisions' as salt beef, pork as hams, and butter, whereas his list of groceries included tea, coffee, sugar, spices and small dried fruits.[8] The trade figures compiled by Porter in his *Progress of the Nation* from 1820 to the 1850s make the same distinction. These two categories were used by the housewife until very recently; she spoke of fetching 'the provisions', meaning butter or margarine, lard, cheese, bacon, eggs, and possibly some cooked meats, and these were served separately in a large grocer's shop at the 'provisions counter'. If she was buying 'groceries' or having them delivered, she meant the sort of dry foods listed by Tooke.

This distinction between the two trades, the grocer and the provision dealer, and their continued use as categories of foodstuffs by traders and customers may also reflect another aspect of these foods. Tea and sugar in particular were luxuries like other groceries such as dried and crystallised fruits; they were not basic elements in the diet until the nineteenth century when tea and sugar in particular began to form an important, even an essential part of the urban diet of all classes. Sweetened tea became the main form of liquid refreshment and a source of comfort and palatibility. This altered the position of the grocer in the food trades, bringing him more central to the housewife's pattern of shopping. This alteration was assisted by the development of other grocery lines, some of which had begun to appear before or about the same time as Indian teas began to be imported in volume in the 1860s to augment and compete with the China teas already on the market.[9] These new lines included various types of processed foods — cornflours, baking powders, dried soups, such as Symingtons' brand, etc.

Our diet is very complex, made up of numerous foods, with even its staple derived from more than one type of grain. Nearly all the ingredients are susceptible to several stages of production and processing either for immediate use or storage. There are also several methods of cooking involving different forms of preparation, of mixing blending, sifting, grating, mincing, drying, etc., which in turn require often specific ingredients such as lard or other types of fat, eggs, milk or some other liquid, and raising agents, to form a mixture of some kind. The rapid growth of an urban population may have stimulated the mass production of some of the requisite ingredients, such as different types of flour and fats, colourings and flavourings to go with them to make bread, cakes, pastry, biscuits, scones and puddings of all types. There were also relatively simple technical processes for pulverising, drying, etc., all sorts of foodstuffs so that they could be sold from a shop as a processed product for further preparation and cooking in the home, such as cornflour, gravy powders, and similar items. Numerous small firms started to manufacture and commercialise a process whereby a raw foodstuff became an ingredient in the family kitchen. Tuckwood, a grocer in Sheffield in the 1860s, was buying dried peas, oatmeal and groats from Symingtons Steam Mills at Market Harborough, and mustard, cocoa, chicory and other commodities from forty different firms including starch and blue from J. & J. Colman's.[10] By the 1880s a grocer in Hull, Jacksons, was buying Wotherspoon's cornflour and also Brown and Polson's brand, Symington's pea flour, borax 'powdered in London', Goodall's custard and egg powders, several brands of tinned milk — Castle's, Swiss and Nestlé's — tinned fruits and Crosse & Blackwell jams, and many other similar items.[11] These extended the stock of the traditional grocer, and also brought into more common use some of his traditional foreign luxuries such as currants and almonds, the latter turned into ground almonds, shelled and split ones, almond paste, and little bottles of almond essence, etc.

It was this kind of quite simple technical revolution, mass producing and semi-processing foodstuffs in common use, together with the rise in tea and sugar consumption, which brought the grocer into focus as the most important food trader for regular family purchases. An alternative revolution in food retailing has sometimes been suggested, pointing to the amalgamation of the trade of the traditional grocer with that of the provision dealer in the second half of the nineteenth century, a development associated with the multiple stores such as Lipton's, Home and Colonial, etc.[12] The revolutionary aspect of these new grocery chains, however, probably lay in their style and organisation of food selling rather than in their range and type of stock. The emergence of a more general grocer or shopkeeper occurred much earlier in the century, either as a result of an amalgamation of the specialist trading of food traders, or of the establishment of a general stores in a locality which served all its food requirements apart from butcher's meat and perhaps fruit and vegetables.[13] The development of this type of store is usually assumed to be associated with the growth of a non-food producing urban-industrial population in this country. How this was done; how customers' demands were defined and met; which goods were supplied and in what form we can only begin to assess. The relationship of the shopkeeper to his trade, both suppliers and consumers, was complex, determined by a number of factors, especially during such a period of rapid change both in economic ideas as well as structure. To attempt to elucidate this is not to deal with 'fringe' activities, but concerns the commercial side of private enterprise industrialisation at its most basic. To do this I have looked first at the organisation of the grocery trade and the emergence of new types of retail outlet, and then secondly at the links between these outlets and their customers.

By the beginning of the nineteenth century in the larger towns there were probably a variety of food traders, of grocers, provision merchants and dealers, specialist tea and coffee dealers, cheesemongers, bakers, and general shopkeepers. They may not all have had fixed shop premises, but movable stalls, barrows and carts, etc. And already there was a certain amount of overlap at the latter stages of the wholesale as well as at the retail end of the trade. The larger towns, ports and market towns in particular offered a sufficient range of incomes and trading potential to sustain a number of traders; wholesalers and retailers specialised in only one or two particular commodities while others were building up a varied and complex trade. Copeman's of Norwich for instance built up a considerable trade as wholesale and retail grocers serving a wide area with imported goods from the end of the eighteenth century onwards.[14] Their range of teas, sugars, different kinds of dried and crystallised fruits, butter and cheeses suggests they catered for the middle and upper income groups. They bought in bulk through Yarmouth from a number of dealers, most of them highly specialised, trading in tea, or sugar, or foreign delicacies, etc. Most of them had warehouses in London, the centre of this import trade, but cheeses and butter came coastwise from the north-west and also via Gainsborough and Hull.

By the middle of the nineteenth century there was still scope for specialisation at the retail end of the trade, with grocers, etc., indicating their speciality on their signs above the shop door and window. They usually carried a wide range of groceries and sometimes provisions too, but their special expertise gave them the particular name they used of grocer, or tea and coffee dealer, etc.; others were cheesemonger, provision dealer, tallow-chandler, oil and colour man, drysalter, Italian warehouseman, etc. The range of goods they carried probably largely depended on the location of their premises. In the main thoroughfares of larger towns there was sufficient trade, and differences in the classes of trade, for a grocer to specialise, attracting particular types of custom by his wares and sales techniques. Others with a shop which served a locality as the main retail source not only of foodstuffs but of other items usually included in their stock goods associated more closely with other trades, such as those of the tallow-chandler — lamp oil, cleaning materials, soaps, candles, brimstone, etc. These were more general shopkeepers; groceries often formed their primary stock-in-trade, but their opportunities for specialisation lay in the sheer range of goods at low prices they carried rather than in particular commodities. They could always extend their range of goods, of foods and other items, as there appeared to be a local demand for them. In this lay the skill, or otherwise, of the local retailer. In poorer districts and in small centres of population there must always have been a tendency for the food retailer with a fixed shop to be a grocer, provision dealer, and general hardware shopkeeper all in one. His may have been the only, or one of a very few, shop premises in the area, serving a variety of needs. Moreover a wide range of goods allowed the shopkeeper to capture all the retail trade available in the locality, and thereby to spread his risks.

In rural areas and isolated villages the shop was probably the centre of more than general retail sales, and became the trading centre for the whole area including the 'putting out' system in domestic industries. Abraham Dent was one of some ten shopkeepers in the market town of

Kirkby Stephen in the eighteenth century, but his range of goods and activities was wide, including sales of foodstuffs, cloth, wines and spirits, etc., and also dealing in knitted stockings.[15] He had large contracts to supply the army with knitted hose, and he organised their knitting by the hand-knitters in the area working in their own homes as an important secondary occupation to agriculture. This is a particularly interesting example of this kind of trader.

All sorts of shopkeepers took on some of the grocer's lines. Jefferys suggests for instance that cheesemongers as retailers – a very old trade – were dying out by the middle of the nineteenth century, except as specialists in the larger urban centres.[16] They were turning themselves more and more into general grocers and provision dealers. Shopkeepers took advantage of the almost daily sales they could make of some items, particularly sugar and tea. But it was not simply a matter of gauging the range of local needs or potential custom, but also of the level of turnover that allowed the carrying of large amounts of stock. This was probably a particular feature of the tea trade. The advent of blended and packaged teas enabled many shopkeepers, large and small, to stock one or two types or brands of tea without having themselves to be a specialist in tea blending and carry large stocks of several teas. Both Horniman and Cassell had been making up small packets of tea in foil-lined paper since the 1850s and even earlier, but it was in the 1880s that pre-packed tea was mass-produced by companies like Lipton's, and the new department stores.[17] David Lewis launched his 'Two-shilling Tea' as part of his development policy for his large department store in Manchester which had already established its place in the clothing trade by selling better goods at the lower end of the price range.[18] As Simmonds stated in the *Practical Grocer* in the early years of this century:

> There are still grocers and tea-dealers who prefer to buy 'originals' – who know their trade and who please their customers better than general blenders can do. But the retailer who has not a fairly large turn-over is out of the running if he tries to blend his own teas – he has to keep too large stocks, and cannot take advantage of the turns of the market unless he has capital . . .
>
> . . . The writer, who was in the trade when China teas only were imported, and has seen the growth and cultivation of Indian and Ceylon and Java teas, is almost dumbfounded as he, in writing this, reflects on the past fifty years of change in methods and prices. Common Congous (wretched stuff), costing 1s., with duty 2s. 2¼d., did not in the old days produce a very choice tea even at 4s. a lb. retail; whereas nowadays a tea very much more drinkable can be and is retailed at 1s. 2d.[19]

Simmonds referred to the 'past fifty years of change in methods and prices'. It was this style of large-scale mass-produced trading that the multiple grocers perfected, as the history of Liptons and Home & Colonial, etc., told by Mathias,[20] illustrates, but was also developed by the Co-operative Wholesale Society.[21] They concentrated on low-priced, readily available, well-displayed general groceries and provisions of an even quality. An important part of their turnover was tea and sugar, the commonest spices of salt and pepper, some pickles and relishes, flour, rice and some dried fruits — a much narrower range of goods, or choices within these categories, than the traditional grocer usually stocked. Within this range there was another foodstuff, mentioned above, which was part of the stock of another trader — flour.

Flour of all kinds and oatmeal for home baking and cereal mixtures became one of the most important items on the shelves of both grocers and general stores. Bakers became largely sellers of the bread and cakes they made; their flour was stocked much more widely by all sorts of retailers. Some grocers set up in business as grocers and flour dealers, as did two men, Carr and Bagshaw in Sheffield in 1845.[22] Their trade was a small one but included three main groups of foodstuffs: flour and other cereals; the goods traditionally associated with the grocer's trade, tea, sugar, dried fruit, coffee and cocoa; and thirdly, 'provisions' or cheese, butter, lard, ham and bacon. They also sold household cleaning materials, candles, etc. This little business went bankrupt, their ledgers in the bankruptcy court files revealing that after a year of trading their customers averaged only four or five a day. We do not know the exact location of the shop, what type of area it attempted to serve, but it was clearly at the other end of the scale from the later CWS stores and those of the multiple grocers. Its history encapsulates the main developments that were taking place in the retail food trades, especially that of the general grocer before the mass-produced commodities like packaged tea began to assist with problems of too small a turnover, etc. Their trade had become that of a general provisions store and grocer, though on too small a scale, but it was the development of this kind of local shop which constituted the retail revolution of the nineteenth century in the food trades — a revolution with some casualties.

The traditional high-class grocer continued to thrive, carrying a very wide range of commodities aimed at the richer customer. The increased output of high-quality British dairy products competing with the foreign Cheddars from Canada,[23] etc., the imported luxury foods and delicacies enabled them to continue to combine the specialist trades of both the grocer and the provision dealer. They stocked Dutch cheeses, and English cheeses bought from specialist dealers, Waterford, Cork and Dublin butter, etc. There were also more mass-produced or processed luxury items by the last decades of the nineteenth century which were often heavily and lavishly advertised. *Law's Grocer's Manual* at the end of the century lists over 360 different types of biscuit for the discriminating grocer keeping his shelves well-stocked with a variety for the customer's individual choice. The advertisements in the *Grocer and Oil Trade Review* diary for some years before this, in 1887, drew attention to a number of specialist items such as Dunn and Hewett's 'lichen islandicus' or Iceland moss cocoa, Van Lookeren, Oyens and Co.'s butterine, Brand's essence of malt sauce, and a silvered page displaying 'Sensation Soap'. There was also pressed on the attention of the retailer a variety of equipment to assist in the preparation of his goods at the back of his shop which he bought in bulk. There were Savage's 'Thorough' fruit cleaning machine, several types of coffee and tea mills, tea mixers, counter scales, store bins, gas coffee roasters, check tills, fancy tea boxes, and everything from shop fittings to paper bags. The retail grocery trade had clearly encouraged the growth of various services and equipment manufactured for its own requirements.

This probably began quite early in the century, and formed part of the general increase in fixed capital equipment and a higher level of investment introduced into retailing and shop premises. These were often quite small items individually, but could add up to a sizeable sum for a shopkeeper to find opening a new shop, or re-equipping his existing premises. Whittock published his *Book of Trades*[24] in the 1830s and recommended that grocers should set up their business with an initial capital of £400 to £600, or about the average capital outlay he suggested for most traders. Many started with far less. London had set the fashion or standards for shop design, especially towards the end of the eighteenth century as a result of the inspiration and work of George Dance the Younger, Clerk of Works to the Corporation of London between 1768 and 1816.[25] As fixed shops, especially in town centres, increased in number and competed with each other, they developed a particular style of trading, using more and more techniques which would now be recognised as 'visual marketing', emphasising large window displays and well-set-out stock in the shop itself. This attracted customers into the shop — either the housewife herself or her servants shopping for her.

This new style of trading became a distinctive feature of modern towns. The growth of towns in the nineteenth century is associated with commerce and trade, especially at the retail level, as well as with particular industries. Fixed shops, often purpose-built, dominated the trading centre of the town supplemented by the weekly market, and by dispersed shops in the outlying districts. In contrast to this the earlier pattern tended to be a central market area with surrounding streets allocated to particular trades for stalls and fixed shops, all geared generally to the market area, almost as a spill-over from it. This is the sort of layout Westerfield suggested had existed in the main market towns some centuries before the modern industrial era, but he also noted that this pattern had begun to break down by the eighteenth century.[26] The increase in incomes and wealth generally as a result of an increase in trade had, he thought, simulated in turn retail trading from fixed shops where goods could be permanently displayed, and a clientele built up. Food traders, perhaps particularly grocers and specialist cheesemongers with perishable goods to sell, were among their number. This relatively slow development in retailing from shop premises in the main market centres was quickened and augmented by the growth in population and rapid industrial urbanisation resulting in the retail revolution of the nineteenth century. This time there was not only an increase in wealth and in the number of wealthy and well-to-do customers among the middle class to be serviced, but also in the number of low income groups of workers.

Jefferys, in placing the revolution in retailing in the latter half of the century, took particular note of the rise in regular working-class incomes, especially post-1870 until the end of the century, on which the multiples and CWS branches based their trade.[27] Alexander has also suggested that the distribution system and its development was determined at least in part by the standard of living and levels of income.[28] There is a danger, however, that an attempt to provide a chronology of developments in the retail grocery and allied trades during urbanisation and industrialisation tends to carry with it the assumption that customer's needs were generally met by shops, itinerant traders and street markets. The type of shop and the stock carried may reflect the income of the residents in the area, but to this extent at least supply and demand are assumed to be in harmony.

Alexander offers some insight into this with his useful calculation of the increase in the number of shops per head in various towns in the first half of the nineteenth century.[29] He selected eleven towns: four very large population centres, five containing some 50,000 people by 1851, and two older centres as cathedral towns, and calculated shop growth rates, that is fixed shop premises, and the ratio of shops to population. He found striking differences between the towns within a general picture of an increasing number of shops as population grew. He offers some interesting comments on this, suggesting that an older established town with a shopping centre may have experienced an increase in the turnover of existing shops, while a new town development from a village base may require a larger net increase in new shops to service a larger population. There may also have been marked variations in the types and sizes of shops depending on the distribution of incomes in the area. Grocers, provision dealers, and general shopkeepers were the largest single category of shop type at mid-century in the towns Alexander looked at, with bakers only marginally less numerous. Of these the highest increase occurred among the general food shopkeepers rather than the better class specialist grocer. Moreover, local multiple trading, or branch shops, were most prominent in the grocery trades.

On the other hand Scola has raised some doubts as to whether the rate of increase in retail food outlets kept pace with the rate of population growth in very large industrial centres like Manchester.[30] There may have been regional, and very local, variations in retail provision whereby some districts were relatively well provided for and others were not. As yet we know too little about the mortality of shops, how far particular shop sites once established remained faithful, so to speak, to a particular trade, so that an area was constantly provided with a grocer's or general store, etc. It has already been suggested that the size of a shop's turnover was crucial to its survival, and determined to some extent the stock carried, but again we are only just beginning to find out the sort of turnover small shops had from the records of bankruptcy cases which caused them to fail. Historical geographers have begun to help us to understand the physical structure of towns and the evolution of districts and suburbs with their services as a result of their analyses of central trading areas and shop dispersal. Considered spatially there may be particular features of a town's development, for instance, which determined its trading centre and the dispersal of shops. In his study of Hull, Shaw found that as the city grew in size the more specialised higher value retail shops were concentrated in the town centre — jewellers, bookshops, watchmakers, etc. — whereas grocers proliferated in the outer growth zone of the town.[31] This is the well-known pattern of dispersal, but he also pointed to the way in which the morphological expansion of Hull was strongly influenced by the river and the dock system. The expansion of the town from its old centre was severely restricted by the development of the docks at the beginning of the nineteenth century, and the residential area was forced out beyond the docks before 1831. This had the effect of isolating the town centre from the main areas of population growth, and stimulating the development of suburban retailing earlier and more effectively than is usually assumed to be the case, and to the detriment of the central trading area of the city.

Similar studies of other towns may reveal other variations or features which throw light on the relationship between the central trading area, the dispersal of shops and the growth of residential suburbs. This kind of spatial analysis can only offer a partial explanation however, leaving many socio-economic questions unanswered — who bought what, for what price, where, from whom and why, for instance. In one form or another it is just these sorts of questions which were being raised and debated from the end of the eighteenth century. It is all too easy to let the history of retailing degenerate into a description of the private trader at work, as he filled the 'niches' in the economy, as Alexander calls them, created by industrialisation and population growth, and waiting to be exploited.[32] Whereas the issues raised by the distribution of goods, especially foodstuffs, were much nearer the bone, and contemporaries involved in the controversies knew it. This was not a short, sharp and therefore neat debate, but one which recurred over a long period of time and over a number of different topics. The main issue was of course free trade, how it should be practised, and the rights of the individual in a free trade situation performing different roles or functions as an entrepreneur, wage-earner, consumer, etc.

The main points of contention about food distribution and supply were: the relaxation of the legislation of earlier centuries controlling wholesaling and retailing defined variously as forestalling, engrossing, etc., and also controlling prices, such as the assize of bread; the development of consumer co-operative trading as an alternative form and ethic of trading; the adulteration of foodstuffs, especially tea and bread, as a trading practice; the payment of wages in kind culminating in legislation against truck; and above all the passing of the 1815 Corn Law and its subsequent repeal. All these raised questions of principle and reflected the major changes taking place in society. To take one example – the freedom of choice of the consumer with the right to exercise his purchasing power as he chose had to be argued through and fought for when it involved wage-earners and their purchases of daily food and other requirements.[33] The problem of 'truck' was discussed, particularly in the 1830s, as a question of the source and price of their foodstuffs and analysed not simply in terms of free trade notions of supply and demand, but in relation to the level of wages, employment opportunities and wage-fund ideas. Hilton has shown how fascinating, and complex, were these ideas surrounding the truck shop.[34] At the practical level they offered employers opportunities for circumventing the standard wage set by collective bargaining, and for raising short-term loans on the inventory of their grocery shop, as well as controlling in some degree the purchasing habits of their workers. At the theoretical level academic or professional economists argued the case for and against high wages, assessing truck as a method of reducing excessive wage payments.[35] To the wage-earner truck shops offered little consumer choice, and reduced his real wages by non-competitive pricing of foodstuffs, etc., below his nominal wages. This occurred in certain areas dominated by particular trades. The 1871 Truck Commission report found a high level of truck payments still operating, despite legislation against such practices, in some colliery districts, iron works, railway construction works, as well as in industries organised on a domestic or workshop basis such as nail-making.[36] Again there were marked regional variations, as there were in the development of cooperative societies with their heavy concentration in the industrial northern countries and in Scotland. At the same time these debates all reflected the way in which the dominant ideas of the period, especially current economic theories, developed out of and were applied to actual situations.

The service sector was controversial, more so probably in the first half of the nineteenth century than at any other time, both the institutions it developed and the ideas it attempted to master. As an integral part of the process of industrialisation and urban growth as it was experienced in this country this was inevitable, but put in this context the history of retailing not only becomes more interesting but also more central to our attempts to understand the changes taking place in society and how they were assessed at the time. The period from about 1780 to 1850 is now beginning to come more into focus, but needs to be looked at more closely still. It was then that the major debates about distribution and trading took place, that the many organisational changes and experiments in types of shops began in response to urban growth and other pressures. By the middle of the century an 'urban diet' had evolved, reflecting to some extent the availability of foodstuffs, as well as dietary habits and income levels. But the interaction between supply and demand was clearly complex, with both acting as dynamic factors, in turn affecting and being affected by the developments in the distribution system. The essential features of the nineteenth century retail food trades may have emerged quite early in the century, but how this was achieved and the debates surrounding this process have still to be explored.

Notes

1. Records in private hands.
2. Particularly various Pitman series, such as 'Common Commodities and Industries' published between 1910 and the 1930s; and specialist studies such as J.M. Walsh, *Tea-Blending as a Fine Art,* Philadelphia, 1896.
3. (J.T. Law), *Law's Grocer's Manual,* Liverpool, 1896; 2nd ed., London, 1902; it is not clear which edition it is in the Cattle papers.
4. For example, F.A. Pearson, *Ticekt and Show Card Designing,* London, 1923.
5. J.A. Rees, *The Grocery Trade, its History and Romance,* 2 vols. bound in one, London, 1932, ii, 260.
6. G. Dodd, *Food of London,* London, 1856.
7. J. Blackman, 'The Development of the Retail Grocery Trade in the Nineteenth Century', *Business History* (1967), ix, no.2, pp.114-5.
8. T. Tooke, *High and Low Prices,* 1823.
9. D. Forrest, *Tea for the British,* London, 1973, esp. Ch.8.
10. Blackman, loc.cit., p.115.
11. Ledgers of the firm of Jacksons in Hull, kindly lent by the firm.
12. J.B. Jefferys, *Retail Trading in Britain, 1850-1950,* London, 1954, pp.1-9, 126-31; and D. Davis, *A History of Shopping,* London, 1966, pp.252-4, 262-3.
13. See the discussion of this in my articles, loc.cit.; 'The Food Supply of an

Industrial Town', *Business History* (1963), v, no.2; and 'Changing Marketing Methods and Food Consumption' in T.C. Barker, J.C. McKenzie and J. Yudkin, *Our Changing Fare*, London, 1966.
14. *Copeman's of Norwich*, Norwich, 1946.
15. T.S. Willan, *Abraham Dent of Kirkby Stephen, an Eighteenth Century Shopkeeper*, Manchester, 1970.
16. Jefferys, op.cit., p.126.
17. Forrest, op.cit., pp.131-4.
18. ibid., pp.175-6.
19. W.H. Simmonds, *The Practical Grocer*, 4 vols., London, 1905, ii, pp.44-5.
20. P. Mathias, *Retailing Revolution*, London, 1967.
21. Jefferys, op.cit., Ch.5.
22. Blackman, 'The Development of the Retail Grocery Trade . . .', loc.cit., pp.115-16.
23. V. Cheke, *The Story of Cheese-Making in Britain*, London, 1959, pp.237-8.
24. N. Whittock *et al.*, *The Complete Book of Trades*, London, 1837.
25. H. Kalman, 'The Architecture of Mercantilism: Commercial Buildings by George Dance the Younger', in P. Fritz and D. Williams (eds.), *The Triumph of Culture: Eighteenth-Century Perspectives*, Toronto, 1972.
26. R.B. Westerfield, *Middlemen in English Business, particularly between 1660-1760*, New Haven, 1915; reprinted New York, 1968, pp.340-47.
27. Jefferys, op.cit., pp.7-9.
28. D. Alexander, *Retailing in England during the Industrial Revolution*, London, 1970, pp.18-25.
29. ibid., Ch.4.
30. R. Scola, paper presented at the Conference of the Urban History Group, Bristol, 4-5 April 1974, 'The Relationship between Food Markets and Shops in Manchester, 1770-1870', and the discussion on that paper: see report of this conference in *Urban History Yearbook, 1975*, pp.31-2.
31. Paper presented by G. Shaw, 'Locational Behaviour of Urban Retailing during the nineteenth century: the example of Kingston-upon-Hull', ibid., p.31.
32. Alexander, op.cit., Ch.1.
33. See some comment on this by C.R. Fay, *Co-operation at Home and Abroad, a description and analysis*, 3rd.ed., London, 1925, pp.272 ff.
34. G.W. Hilton, *The Truck System*, Cambridge, 1960.
35. W. Cunningham's discussion of this is interesting, *The Growth of English Industry and Commerce in Modern Times*, part II, *Laissez Faire*, pp.737-45.
36. Hilton, op.cit., pp.131-49.

13 J. LYONS & CO. LTD. : CATERERS & FOOD MANUFACTURERS, 1894 TO 1939[1]

D.J. RICHARDSON

The hotel and catering trades form one of the country's largest employers of labour. The creation of this industry over the last century has been the result of a complex equation involving increased affluence and changing social habits. This paper recounts the early history of one of the best-known catering companies, J. Lyons & Co. Ltd., with the purpose of filling at least some of the gaps in our knowledge about the history of catering as a form of food distribution. In the course of analysing Lyons' experience some reference is naturally made to the environment in which the company operated. This is not an easy task because, in common with other distributive trades, catering has long been characterised by the existence of a multitude of small traders who have left few records of their business activities. Indeed, independent operators still dominate the trade because there is a high premium on personal service and local managerial control. It is recognition of this factor which gives particular interest to the way in which Lyons succeeded in applying multiple trading techniques to catering. The rapid growth of the company's teashop chain was supported by food production at its headquarters, Cadby Hall, and in the 1920s this food manufacturing side of the business was dramatically increased by wholesaling tea, ice cream and cake to a vast army of retail agents. Thus Lyons plays a doubly significant role in the history of diet: firstly as a specialist in the service of food in catering establishments and secondly as a large-scale food manufacturer. Since the prosperity of the latter phase of Lyons' history was linked with the fortunes of the independent retailer it provides an interesting contrast with the firm's own multiple expansion, as well as a useful reflection of more general features of food distribution in the period. Lyons' first teashop opened in Piccadilly in 1894. The history of the early years of the firm's life needs to be seen firstly in the context of the growth of Victorian and Edwardian London, and secondly against the familiar background of general expansion of the service industries at that time.[2] The dramatic rise of the multiples in the retail food trade established a pattern which was followed in many respects by catering. In short, Lyons' early activities need to be firmly located in the retailing revolution.

In the middle of the nineteenth century London was badly served by catering outlets at all levels. Clubs like the Reform provided meals for the wealthy, as did the chop houses, but both groups were primarily male preserves; ladies were not acceptable in the former and the latter were not acceptable to ladies. The provision of catering facilities for the metropolitan masses, or even for the growing band of office workers, remained rudimentary, and largely based on the public-house. As the demand for catering services grew, so traditional outlets were the first to expand. Many taverns, for example, began to provide cooked vegetables and cooking facilities for their customers, who purchased their steaks and chops at local butchers. A contemporary described a number of such places within a hundred yards radius of the Royal Exchange,[3] as well as mentioning the existence of a collection of dining rooms, eating-houses, oyster rooms and alamode beef shops, many of which served poor quality food in unhygienic surroundings at high prices. Travelling salesmen also expanded their business in the buoyant catering market of the 1860s. The activities of these characters were immortalised in the legends surrounding the Flying Pieman; they were carefully analysed by Mayhew in Volume 1 of his *London Labour and the London Poor*.[4] Mayhew looked at the activities of thirty-three classes of such salesmen, from the street-sellers of pea soup and hot eels to travellers selling ham sandwiches, baked potatoes and boiled puddings. He estimated that four thousand people were engaged in such refreshment vending, that £203,115 was spent annually on their wares, and that the capital employed in the industry came to the amazingly precise figure of £9,077.12*s.* 5*d*.[5]

As the pace of change accelerated in the last quarter of the century so these traditional outlets were joined by new caterers, many of whom offered better food in more pleasant surroundings. The Post Office Directories list 345 Dining Rooms in London in 1848. Thirty years later there were four hundred Dining Rooms and three hundred Refreshment Rooms, while by 1902 there were over one thousand Dining Rooms and eight hundred Refreshment Rooms and Cafes. Even disregarding the undoubted improvement in quality which took place, it is still obvious from this indicator that there was a considerable growth in the number of catering outlets in operation, an increase which was a direct response to the growth of London, the large-scale development of commuting, and rising standards of living. The most important developments in the trade between 1875 and 1900 took place along two well-defined lines of new catering enterprise: temperance catering and commercial catering.

Temperance catering was a fascinating movement which spread well outside London. It grew from temperance reformers' realisation that although their campaign for prohibition of alcohol might be futile, practical ways might be found in which the drink problem could be mitigated. Thus, in the 1870s several temperance societies began developing coffee public-houses in which people could enjoy all the comfort, warmth and social life which they sought in a traditional public-house while drinking tea and coffee rather than beer and spirits.

In many cases these coffee houses, with their bars and inn signs, were intended to be exact replicas of their alcoholic counterparts. Nothing could be more appealing to the Victorian reforming mind than the combination of private profit and social gain represented by the coffee taverns, and the movement grew. By 1879 there were a hundred such establishments in London alone, while five years later there were 232 limited liability companies in the country owning 667 coffee public-houses besides 646 independent institutions.[6] The operation of many of these undertakings was plagued by inefficiency; general incompetence which allowed the movement to drift towards disaster in the 1880s. The reasons for this were simple. Firstly, it was a bad misjudgement to assume that working men went to public-houses to enjoy the social life without caring whether they drank any alcohol. Secondly, while a person might drink eight or nine pints of beer in an evening, two cups of coffee were quite sufficient. As a leading figure in the movement, Arthur Jepson, put it: 'Persons do not require to be constantly wetting their throats with coffee and tea.'[7] High rents, bad siting and amateurish management all played their parts, as did the poor quality of refreshment provided in some coffee houses. A contemporary scathingly remarked that the coffee taverns were 'gaining an unenviable notoriety for a beverage that is not only cheap but nasty'.[8]

As a result of these difficulties of the early 1880s many coffee tavern proprietors were forced to reform or re-direct their activities, creating the nucleus of what could be recognised as a catering business. Some offered entertainment as a means of inducing customers to stay and drink more coffee; others began to provide food as an attraction or as a profit-making activity. Some multiplied their branches and sought the economies of backward integration; a few sought to escape the dilemma of working-class catering by raising prices, so widening the gap between costs and receipts. There was a distinct change from a movement to an industry, the most important feature of this recasting being the emergence of two sizeable companies, Lockharts and Pearce & Plenty. Common to both was the idea that philanthropy without commercial success was worthless. Lockharts had a very limited menu of cocoa, coffee and tea, sandwiches, sausages, Melton Mowbray pies, pastry and bread, and concentrated on good sites. Pearce & Plenty's success was largely due to the enterprising personality of John Pearce himself. The motto and operational principles of his dining rooms were explicit if rather basic: 'Quality, Economy, Despatch'. The lunchtime menu was steak pudding and potatoes 5*d.*, two sausages and potatoes 4*d.* with tea at 1*d.* or 1½*d.*[9] By 1893 Lockharts had a chain of fifty coffee rooms and Pearce & Plenty ran twenty dining rooms.

The emergence of one or two efficient multiple operations against the background of a trade dominated by independent units was also the pattern in commercial catering. Indeed, with the growing emphasis on the commercial viability of coffee taverns and cocoa rooms there was only a narrow dividing line between these reforming societies, and the growing number of companies which were providing light refreshments with no other motive than to make a profit. The Aerated Bread Company and the Express Dairy both developed 'milk and bun' shops as an adjunct to their main trade, while such companies as Spiers and Pond, Slaters and Gattis also became active in the business. By 1893 the Aerated Bread Company had sixty cafes, while the last three companies also became operators of high-class restaurants. In this field they were quickly joined by the large new hotels which had begun to trade in London from the 1860s, offering dinners in surroundings of dazzling luxury, and by a new breed of restaurants such as the Gaiety, the Holborn and the Criterion. A piece of doggerel from *The Bat* of January 1886 gives some of the atmosphere of the changes occurring:

> One day he travelled up to town on dissipation bent
> And to the Albion itself at supper time he went.
> He sought the famous hostelry that's close to Drury Lane;
> He walked inside the Albion, he stared, he stared again.
> He staggered back surprised and then he murmured, soft and low,
> In accents of astonishment 'Well, here's a pretty go'
> Here's the sawdust gone completely, here's a carpet rich and thick,
> Here's journalists a-supping and not demanding tick,
> Here's a very showy tablecloth, a fork that's free from dirt,
> And a waiter young and lively, with no gravy on his shirt,
> Here's a general conspiracy my sentiments to hurt
> For dissolving an old partnership of genius and dirt.
> That rustic homeward hied him and was never after heard,
> To say in praise of Spiers and Pond another blessed word.
> They'd trampled on his sympathies, they'd actually been,
> And made the stuffy Albion respectable and clean.

It was in this period of expansion in the catering trade that Lyons was born; it was in the atmosphere of respectability and cleanliness that the new company made its mark by joining the ranks of the multiple caterers.

Catering

Although Lyons was incorporated as a public company in 1894 it had been in operation as a contract exhibition caterer since the Newcastle Exhibition of 1887. The business was directed by two families, the Salmons and the Glucksteins, so closely bonded by marriage as to form one family group. They were already well-known for a thriving tobacco business called Salmon & Gluckstein, and when Montague Gluckstein sought to diversify the family's interests by starting catering it was decided that a new name should be chosen to avoid confusion with the existing business. On his travels as a cigar salesman, Montague had observed the poor quality of refreshments at exhibitions, and the Newcastle Exhibition offered a suitable opportunity for the family to test market its catering ideas. Montague's brother Isidore was engaged to a girl who had a distant relation running a stall at the Liverpool Exhibition. Since his experience in the exhibition business matched the brothers' requirements, he was approached and offered a leading role in the venture, that of giving it his name. That stallholder was Joseph Lyons, later to become chairman of the public company and popularly credited with the development of Joe Lyons teashops as a national institution. Nevertheless, the organising genius of the firm was really Montague Gluckstein, ably assisted by his brother Isidore, and later by his cousin, Alfred Salmon.

Once the idea of a teashop chain had been initiated it is clear that the family's experience of shop siting and personal service in the tobacco trade was extremely useful. Moreover, their accumulated prosperity was important in allowing them to experiment with new ideas and support infant projects. The price reduction they had offered on their tobacco products had been given ample publicity — their favourite slogan was 'The more you smoke, the more you save' — and they were ready to invest substantial amounts in creating a catering business. When the Newcastle Exhibition closed prematurely, Lyons continued to run their tea pavilion, hiring a Hungarian orchestra at a cost of £150 a week to provide the entertainment. Their more cautious contemporaries were scandalised at this audacious outlay on the prospective profits of light refreshments, but the exercise was very successful, and the Lyons catering enterprise had begun.

Further catering contracts were successfully served until, seven years after the Newcastle Exhibition, the first Lyons teashop was opened. The very short time interval before others were opened leaves no doubt that Lyons intended to operate the shops as a chain. This view is supported by the fact that all the teashops were uniform in price and decoration. The menu was lighter and more sophisticated in its range of choice than those of the Pearce & Plenty or Lockhart depots and this, combined with superior decoration, appealed to ladies shopping, to clerks who would return home for a hot evening meal (as opposed to Pearce & Plenty clients who had their main meal at midday) and above all, at the turn of the century and after the First World War, to the growing army of London typists. Respectability, quality, cheapness, speed and cleanliness became the Lyons watchwords. The guiding commercial principle was that of multiples in every trade, that of a small profit on a large turnover. In the 1920s the profit on a full-scale meal in a teashop was reckoned to be less than ¼d.

Some firms engaged in temperance catering, some in commercial catering and some in exhibition catering. One of the early strengths of Lyons was the fact that it crossed these simple divisions. It started in exhibition catering, went on to exploit the temperance market with its chain of teashops and entered the sphere of commercial catering with its Corner Houses and restaurants. The first of these high-class restaurants was the Trocadero, opened in 1896 on a site in Piccadilly which *The Caterer* described as being 'the centre of pleasure-seeking London'.[10] Although the Trocadero was opened at a time when the teashop chain was being established it is clear that the opening of the teashops had little or no direct bearing on the initiation of plans for the Trocadero; the latter was in a completely different class of catering enterprise. The external stimulus to the growth of the teashops was the general improvement in standards of living and the increasingly large numbers of people forced to spend long periods away from home. The external stimulus to the Trocadero, the demand factor, was less a case of changes in economic factors than a change in social habits amongst the wealthy. There was a noticeable increase in the fashion of dining out, and, as part of this, a slow acceptance that it was now respectable for accompanied ladies to dine out and even to entertain guests at a restaurant:

> Men don't dine at their clubs nowadays; they go with their wives or the wives of others to partake of the Restaurant Dinner. These Restaurant Dinners are comparatively recent institutions, so to speak, having come into vogue during the last few years, but they have become almost, if not altogether, the greatest feature of the Night Side of London high life.[11]

The *Penny Illustrated* in its glowing report on the Trocadero was quite sure of its success 'since it has now become the fashion for families to dine and give parties at a restaurant, much to the comfort of many housewives'.[12] The manager of the Trocadero, Mr. Alfred Salmon, besides providing novel features such as a *table d'hôte* inclusive of wine for as little as five shillings, and entertainment in the form of a regimental band, pandered to this respectability. A written code stipulated that 'strange ladies', whether alone or in pairs, were not to be admitted, or if by some oversight they had been let in, they were to be secluded by screens from the public gaze.

The trading success of the Trocadero was quickly consolidated by the Throgmorton Restaurant, opened by Lyons in 1900 directly opposite the Stock Exchange. An early Board minute records the decision to incorporate a high-class restaurant and a light refreshment depot on the same site, and the *Weekly Despatch* noted that:

City clerks will be as well served for the common or garden 'bob' as the more aristocratic half-sovereign, and whatever you have will bear the hall mark of good quality.[13]

The Throgmorton is important because it explicitly sought to exploit both sections of the catering market — the demand deriving from changing social habits and that created by the growth of London as a commercial centre. Because it served a specific geographical area it is also possible to sketch the Throgmorton's position in the changing catering trades. In the earlier part of the nineteenth century the Stock Exchange was fed by three coffee houses, a bun stall, Moth's and Elphinstone's eating houses and Horace Potter's Restaurant. Mabey's, Porch's and Birch's, three chop houses, linked the period of sanded floors and the palatial Throgmorton:

> Lyons have deliberately killed the old-fashioned Chop-house keeper with his dirty kitchen, horse-box cubicles, cracked crockery, discoloured pewter cutlery, fuddled waiters and stiff prices. He is dead and no one will mourn his loss, for he was a disgrace to the City and a marvel to all foreigners who were taken by cynical friends to see how the British person ate his lunch . . . And what is more the patron's bill will not be higher than when he patronised the pre-historic Chop-house round the Corner.[14]

Lyons' interests in high-class licensed catering represented by the Trocadero and the Throgmorton were expanded by the opening of the first Corner House in 1909. The period between 1895 and 1914 was also one of rapid growth of the teashop chain, with a new shop opening on average every six weeks. The company was now expanding at the expense of its competitors. Pearce & Plenty and Lockharts had become direct competitors in the middle-class teashop market by launching two new companies, the British Tea Table and the Ideal Restaurants, but their challenge was never dangerous, and in the former case became distinctly weaker when John Pearce resigned from his Board in 1905, after acrimonious discussions with his fellow directors. At about the same time the ABC became involved in an unsuccessful tobacco venture and Spiers & Pond were losing money heavily in an attempt to build up a chain of hotels. Meanwhile Lyons continued to acquire valuable London sites and began to open provincial teashops.

The First World War caused little change in the competitive structure of the catering trade, and Lyons emerged in the inter-war period as the country's largest caterer. Its catering fleet now consisted of two hundred and fifty teashops, three Corner Houses, each capable of seating up to three thousand people, and its flagship, the Trocadero. Lyons waitresses, the nippys, were accepted as 'the symbol of public service', and the company had produced a slogan which became used nationally — 'Where's George? Gone to Lyonch.' The firm's catering had become part of the social scene, familiar to Londoners and visitors alike. When millions visited the Wembley Exhibition it was Lyons who fed them, when eight thousand people sat down to a Masonic banquet in 1925 it was Lyons who dined them, and when guests at Buckingham Palace garden parties ate strawberries and cream it was Lyons who served them.

Despite the increased scope of the business the teashop chain was the basis of the Lyons' catering activities. It had been conceived as a multiple operation and this remained the key feature of its organisation: standardised units drawing all their supplies, including cooked food, from Cadby Hall. Within this trading framework it is possible to identify three key factors contributing to the successful expansion of the chain.

Firstly, there was an unswerving belief in providing the public with consistently good value at popular prices. The cups of tea sold in the shops were produced from the finest blends, the most popular meal in the teashops, roast beef and two vegetables, cost only 10*d.*, and a *table d'hôte* lunch at a Corner House cost as little as 1*s.* 6*d.* Secondly, particular attention was paid to acquiring only the best trading sites. Thirdly, the company evolved an advanced system of portion control and elaborate checking which ensured the elimination of waste and pilfering. This was possible when a situation of labour surplus provided ample supplies of clerical staff at low cost:

> Major Salmon describes another clue to Lyon's success as being 'up to date' commonsense methods directed to the vigorous elimination of wastage. To this end has been built up a most elaborate checking system, whereby the smallest individual transaction is subjected to careful analytical scrutiny.
>
> As part of this the waitresses check, which the customer gives up at the paybox after ordering a meal at a Lyons restaurant or teashop, goes through something like eight pairs of hands at Cadby Hall and stage by stage it is classified, checked, analysed, credited to the waitresses and recorded in its proper place as a unit of the business done that day by that depot. If anywhere a leakage has occurred it is detected within a few hours and the individual responsible among all the twenty-two thousand employees of the company is known.[15]

Lyons was extremely efficient at applying advanced methods of control in a persistent effort to reduce costs while retaining a high level of service. However, as the teashop chain grew, it inevitably became more difficult to maintain the degree of flexibility which was required in a market characterised by rapidly changing social habits. Shorter working weeks meant fewer customers for the breakfast and high tea business. Tea in the office clearly had an effect on morning and afternoon trade. Could these be compensated for by increased numbers at lunch-time, or by greater custom from shoppers? How far should a large firm adapt its business to passing fads, such as the milk-bar craze of the mid-1930s? All these posed possible difficulties for any caterer and real problems for Lyons which remained reluctant to increase prices. By the 1930s the profitability of the teashops had begun to decline significantly. The Corner Houses continued to make sound profits, but the popular image of Lyons as a company based predominantly on catering became increasingly misleading. By 1939 a large proportion of the firm's profits was already derived from food manufacturing and wholesaling.

Food Manufacturing

Retail sales of Lyons' goods at the cash desks of the teashop had been made from an early stage in the firm's history. As the business grew, so the range of products increased, and the inclusion of a front shop for such sales became a characteristic feature of the Corner Houses as well as the teashops. In response to public demand some tea was sold by post by the end of the nineteenth century and door-to-door deliveries of bread and cakes were also made at the same time. Sales continued from the cash counters of the catering outlets, but this retailing phase was otherwise short-lived, especially for tea, for which a large-scale agency business was in operation by 1904. Similar wholesale methods were applied to ice cream and to bread and cakes in the early and mid-1920s respectively, and by 1939 Lyons was established as a large-scale food manufacturer and distributor. The company sold its tea through two hundred thousand agents, produced three and a half million gallons of ice cream, and baked sixty-three thousand tons of bread and cake each year.

A key element in the origin of each of the food manufacturing and wholesale parts of the business was the company's catering requirement. Skills of tea buying and blending and bakery manufacture were developed as the catering business expanded, and it was natural that an enterprising business should develop them in a wider field. Montague Gluckstein saw the potential for a wholesale tea operation and he was directly responsible for employing an extremely able sales manager, G.A. Pollard, to direct the sales force. Pollard dominated this side of the business throughout much of the inter-war period, while the overall control of the Tea Department passed to Montague's nephew Harry Salmon, probably the ablest of the business's second-generation members. Maurice Salmon, Harry's brother, was responsible for the ice cream, cake and bread departments, similarly assisted by a dynamic sales manager, W.I. Brown. Maurice had disliked his training in the catering and hotel business and as a result had been discounted by the family, but in the 1920s he began to demonstrate great skill at organising factory production. By the late 1930s his single-minded dedication to this side of the business had had such successful results that his plans for expansion were rarely challenged by his family, and the Cadby Hall site became crammed with new factory buildings. The replacement of one generation by another is probably the biggest problem for any family business. Lyons was unusual in the ease with which the founders were replaced not only by men of similar calibre but by those who were active and highly successful in the development of new fields of business; the company was rather more typical in that this was the result of good fortune rather than good planning.

Lyons was by no means the first company to sell packet tea, but by the inter-war period it shared the lead in this growing business with Brooke Bond. The ice cream and packaged cake trade were more original and the company played an important role in creating markets for these new convenience foods. Maurice Salmon was a shrewd observer of the American food industry and his development of the Cadby Hall site drew heavily on American ideas, both in the broad appreciation of the potential of mass production of food and in the application of specific factory techniques and processes. Special recipes were devised by the Lyons laboratories and factory buildings were specially designed by Lyons engineers to cope with production on a scale hitherto unknown. Visitors to the site were astonished to learn that the daily production of swiss rolls could be measured in miles.

Mass production methods lowered food costs but also required efficient systems for mass distribution. The sale of tea followed a conventional pattern; transport by rail to a series of depots and then by salesmen's motor vans to individual agents. In the 1920s and 1930s efforts were made to widen the scope of the Tea Agents Departments by selling other grocery lines, such as toffee, custard powder and tomato ketchup. In most cases these products faced fierce competition from acknowledged brand leaders and apart from coffee and coffee extract (Bev) the development of grocery lines was unsuccessful. The perishability of cakes and ice cream meant that a quicker distribution was essential, and the company used the railways for this purpose. Goods were packed at Cadby Hall, taken to the nearby Addison Road station and then consigned to the railways for delivery to retail outlets. Lyons' salesmen could telephone orders to Cadby Hall one evening and expect delivery of the goods to the agent the next morning. In any event delivery by the railway companies within twenty-four hours was guaranteed.

The creation of an efficient way of delivering goods was one part of a general commitment to freshness, cleanliness and good value which was regarded by Lyons' directors as being a necessary element in the success of a branded goods business. Providing good value to the customers meant cutting the agent's profit margin to the minimum, persuading him that he would be compensated by a large turnover. Lyons sought to provide the independent retailer with a product which was highly competitive with that of the multiples. In addition the company created an environment in which it performed many of the functions which in the late nineteenth century had been the preserve of the multiples. The goods were heavily promoted, particularly at point of sale, and regular deliveries allowed shopkeepers to ensure the freshness of the products they were selling.

Conclusion

The operation of the Lyons teashop chain fits well into the picture of increasing importance of multiple trading in the late nineteenth century. By contrast, the company's food manufacturing and wholesale business in the inter-war period depended on the large potential market for branded goods amongst independent retailers. This latter phase involved a process of interdependence because small traders' access to nationally branded goods such as Lyons tea, and to new products, such as packaged cake and ice cream, was an important element of strength in competing with the multiples. Traditional retailing barriers were broken down as Lyons opened up large numbers of new outlets. For example, while a bakery trade journal in 1929 lamented the increased cake trade being done by grocers, a contemporary journal urged its bakery members to widen the scope of their own businesses:

> There is no doubt that the ice cream brick has come to stay ... Most keen confectioners nowadays realise the value of ice cream as a side line.[16]

Lyons' prosperity in the inter-war years was therefore due increasingly to its food manufacturing business rather than to its catering interests. The shifting emphasis of the business occurred without a break in continuity because the company's enterprising management had achieved the prime condition for success — adaptation to general economic and social conditions.

Notes

1. This paper is based on a history of J. Lyons & Co. Ltd. which is currently being prepared. I am grateful to the Board of Lyons for their permission to publish it, and to Professor T.C. Barker for his help and advice.
2. Cf. J.B. Jefferys, *Retail Trading in Britain 1850–1950*, 1954, and P. Mathias, *Retailing Revolution*, 1967.
3. Knight's *London*, 1843, Chapter XCV.
4. H. Mayhew, *London Labour and the London Poor, Vol. 1*, 1964, pp.166-226.
5. ibid., p.166.
6. *The Coffee Public-House News*, November 1879, p.227, and *The Coffee Tavern Guide*, 1884.
7. *The Coffee Public-House News*, May 1884, p.57.
8. ibid.
9. *The Caterer*, 15 February 1893.
10. *The Caterer*, 15 October 1896.
11. R. Machray, *The Night Side of London*, 1902, p.69.
12. *The Penny Illustrated Paper*, 4 October 1896.
13. *The Weekly Despatch*, 7 October 1900.
14. *The Empire*, 10 October 1900.
15. *The Hotel Review*, October 1922.
16. *The British & Foreign Confectioner & Baker*, 1 May 1927.

14 THE DEVELOPMENT OF THE FOOD-CANNING INDUSTRY IN BRITAIN DURING THE INTER-WAR PERIOD

JAMES P. JOHNSTON

During the early twenties the canning of food in Britain was still a small-scale and experimental business. Canned foods, however, were not new to the British public. Since long before the First World War, imports of a wide variety of canned products had been catering for a steadily increasing demand. The war itself did much to convince many people of the merits of canned foods, and after 1918 imports of these products assumed substantial proportions. Imports of canned fruits preserved in syrup, for example, which had averaged 534,000 cwts. over the period 1909-13[1] increased rapidly after the war to reach 2,100,000 cwts. by 1924.[2] Canned beef imports increased from an average of 534,000 cwts. over the period 1909-13 to 966,000 cwts. in 1924[3] and similarly imports of canned fish, canned vegetables and condensed milk all increased rapidly to stand at 1,065,000 cwts., 718,000 cwts.[4] and 2,182,000 cwts. respectively in 1924.[5]

Undoubtedly, therefore, a rapidly expanding market existed for a wide range of canned foods. By 1924, however, the share of British canners in this market was, as yet, relatively small. According to the census of production for 1930, the share of the home market held by British products in 1924 was as follows:

   Canned Meat – 15%
   Canned Fish – 1.8%
   Canned Vegetables – 5.1%
   Canned Fruit (in syrup) – 2.7%[6]
   Condensed Milk – 23.9%[7]

Clearly, the scope for expansion in the British canning industry was enormous. However, canners in this country were faced with a number of problems in the fields of technology, organisation, finance and marketing. Until these could be overcome there was little hope of the British industry gaining anything but a minute share of the market dominated by importing produce.

Around the mid-twenties, however, interest in the potentialities of canning as a commercial venture, so interested parties. This meeting to a meeting between a number of interesting parties. This meeting represented the first determined bid to come to grips with the problems confronting British canners. Among those present were several canners who were already operating under the existing difficult conditions, a number of businessmen interested in taking up canning, suppliers of raw materials such as fruit and vegetables, members of the Welsh tinplate industry, representatives of the tin box manufacturing industry and some research scientists who had been working on technical problems involved in the canning process. The initiative to arrange this meeting had come from the Ministry of Agriculture and Fisheries, whose interest stemmed from the belief that, on the one hand, the expansion of the British canning industry would be of some assistance to the agricultural sector by providing another outlet for agricultural produce and, on the other hand, might go some way towards reducing the increasing flow of imports. The outcome of the meeting was the formation of the National Food Canning Council under the Chairmanship of Sir Edgar Jones, a leading figure in the Welsh tinplate industry. The object of this body was to co-ordinate the activities of the various interests associated with the canning industry and to promote the British industry by means of national propaganda. It was also agreed that all technological problems should be dealt with at Camden Research Station in Gloucestershire.

From this time on the industry began to expand rapidly. By 1927 there were 27 factories in England and Wales, engaged in fruit and vegetable canning alone. By 1931 this number had risen to 59,[8] and by 1933 to 74.[9] In Scotland, where the main activity was fruit canning, there were already five factories in operation by 1931,[10] and by 1934 this number had risen to nine.[11]

Table I: *Output of Principal Products of British Canning Industry 1924-35 (000 Cwts.)*

	1921	1930	1935
Meat	172*	364*	406*
Fish	151	140	173
Vegetables	40	314†	1213†
Fruit	117	315	466
Condensed Milk	766	875	2975
Soups	–	130	234

Source: Census of Production 1930, 1935.

*includes meat extracts. Not separately distinguished for 1924. For 1930 – 98,000 cwts. For 1935 – 91,000 cwts.

†Output of bottled vegetables included. For 1930 – 9,000 cwts. For 1935 – 9,000 cwts.

Table I shows the extent of the increases in output of the various branches of the industry between the three census years 1924, 1930 and 1935. The rapid growth of the late twenties is immediately apparent, especially in the canning of fruit, vegetables and meat. During the thirties, however, there were signs that some branches of the canning industry were having difficulty in sustaining their initial impetus. Persistent over-production, price-cutting, and stock-dumping pointed to the existence of serious weaknesses in the market for British canned produce. The fact is that the rapid expansion of the late twenties, while reflecting the great progress being made in the technological sphere, also brought to light new problems in other areas which seriously retarded the development of the industry during the thirties. The purpose of this paper is to examine some of the more important aspects in the development of the British canning industry during the inter-war period, focusing on the nature and extent of the major problems confronting canners in this country. Only in this way can an adequate measure of the overall achievement be gained.

Technology

During the early twenties, the handful of companies engaged in canning activities in Britain operated under serious technological difficulties. The industry at this stage, according to one report, was 'hampered by lack of men with an adequate knowledge of canning processes and machinery, and by the high costs inseparable from small and more or less experimental undertakings'.[12] The alleviation of this situation came in two ways after 1925: first, by the intensive investigation of a wide range of technical problems related to the canning process, carried out in several food research institutions in Britain, and secondly, by the transmission of the experience and technical resources of some leading firms in the huge American canning industry, through agreements with several British can and machinery manufacturers.

By far the most important of these research establishments in Britain was the Fruit and Vegetable Preservation Research Station, at Chipping Camden in Gloucestershire. Initially established to investigate ways of conserving home-produced foods during the First World War, this research station, after 1918, lapsed into a centre for summer courses on the domestic preservation of food. However, the appointment of two full-time researchers in 1923 transformed the role of the station. Both these men had had previous connections with industry, and having surveyed the possible directions their work could take, they decided that great potential lay in the as yet little exploited field of canning on a commercial scale. From the outset, the work of the station was of a practical nature. The researchers devoted their attention to the solution of actual problems confronting British canners. As the industry developed in the late twenties, Camden Research Station became the focal point of research and advice on cannery problems. Trials to find the best varieties of produce for canning were carried out. The problems of corrosion in tins and the question of metal contamination in canned foods were investigated. In 1928, Camden provided the industry with a method of preserving the greenness in vegetables, and later gave birth to the idea of the 'processed pea', which was to become the most popular of all canned vegetables. These are just a few examples of the invaluable assistance given to the industry by the researchers at Camden. The Station kept in close contact with the firms in the industry, giving advice on a wide range of subjects, including even factory-layout costing. This liaison was strengthened by the establishment of a technical advisory committee, consisting of members of the station and many of the top technical men from the major firms. In 1926, the station answered 97 commercial enquiries relating to cannery problems. By 1931, this number had risen to 518,[13] and in 1933, the figure was 1,007.[14] The work of the Station was widened further when it was given the task of inspecting samples of canned goods under the National Mark Scheme, which was extended to canned fruit and vegetables in 1930, in an attempt to introduce standards of quality to the industry.

So closely, in fact, did the Research Station at Camden become involved in the development of the canning industry in Britain, that in 1930, the government decided that it should, henceforward, be financed by the firms using its services. Under a new contributory scheme, the canners themselves began to foot the bill. Some indication of the value placed on its work is the fact that by the end of 1932, 100 firms allied to the industry were contributing to the station's running costs.[15] Besides Camden Research Station, although of less importance, investigations in the field of canning began at the Low-Temperature Research Station at Cambridge, and at Hannah Dairy Research Station, which were both under the aegis of the Department of Scientific and Industrial Research. In addition, valuable work was being done by the International Tin Research and Development Council.

The practical assistance given to the canning industry by the work of Camden and other institutions was complemented to a great extent by the wealth of knowledge and technical expertise gained by those involved in the long-established American canning industry. The transmission of this knowledge was an important feature of the development of the British canning industry. In the field of canning machinery, American influence was initially of paramount importance. The fact is that before 1930, all of the machinery in use in British canneries was imported from America. By this date, however, British engineers were awakening to the possibilities in this sphere and were soon turning out a wide range of machinery, much of it, significantly, similar in design to the American equipment. This, however, was not the end of American involvement in the British market for canning machinery. Indeed, in an attempt to maintain a foothold in this market, the Food Machinery Corporation of America concluded an agreement with a British firm, Mather and Platt Ltd., in 1932. Under the terms of this agreement a company was formed known as Food Machinery (Mather and Platt) Ltd. From 1932, the range of machinery made at Mather and Platt's Manchester works was extended to include machinery made to the designs of the Food Machinery Corporation. In return, the experience and technical resources of the latter company were placed at the disposal of Mather and Platt.[16]

American companies also played a major role in the field of can-making. The maintenance of an adequate supply of good quality cans was, in fact, one of the earliest and most pressing problems confronting canners in this country. Despite the enterprising efforts of some tin box manufacturers, notably G.H. Williamsons of Worcester, who in 1927 installed a semi-automatic can-making plant, it was a sad fact that by 1929, according to one observer, 'the absence of good cans at an economic price (was) hampering the development of the British industry'. The same writer goes on to say that, 'in spite of the fact that can-makers in Britain obtained supplies of tin plates at prices roughly 15 per cent less than makers in the United States, the prices of cans in Britain are from 25 to 30 per cent more than those ruling on the other side of the Atlantic. This in part arises from the large quantity of defective cans — placed authoritatively at up to 25 per cent — turned out by British makers. This contrasts with approximately 1 per cent of wasters in the United States.'[17] It is debatable whether can-makers were wholly to blame for the excessive number of defective cans. There had been many complaints during the twenties about the quality of British tinplates, particularly from merchants engaged in their export. British tinplate producers, for their part, alleged that the practice, common among merchants, of re-sorting and re-grading tinplates to their own advantage, provided the basis of many of the complaints. However, Walter Minchinton, in his study of the British tinplate industry, pointed out that in 1928 the chairman of one of the leading companies in the industry reported, that, as a result of an appeal by the Joint Industrial Council, quality had 'improved'[18]: the implication is unmistakable. At any rate, from a purely technical viewpoint British tinplate production methods were by the early thirties becoming increasingly antiquated by international standards. Indeed, it was not until 1938, that the first strip-mill, the basis of modern tinplate manufacture, was completed in Britain. By this time there were already 28 in operation in the United States.[19]

The entry of the Metal Box Company Ltd. into the can-making

business marks the beginning of the end of can supply problems. This company took over G.H. Williamsons, and in 1931 opened a large new can-making factory at Worcester with a capacity of 1,200 cans per minute. The directors of Metal Box then concluded an agreement with the Continental Can Company, one of America's two leading can-making concerns. This agreement ensured Metal Box the use of the experience and technical resources of the American company. Following on this, the other leading American can-making firm, American Can Company Ltd., attempted to infiltrate the British market, by concluding an agreement with the newly-floated British Can Company under the terms of which, the former agreed to supply 'on satisfactory terms[20] machinery and equipment together with expert assistance and information'. This infiltration was brought to an abrupt halt by the aggressive policy of the Metal Box Company which by the end of 1931 had become so well-entrenched in the British market that it was able to take over the British Can Company. Under the terms of the takeover agreement all the American directors on the board of the British Can Company resigned from their positions. The directors of Metal Box then proceeded to conclude an agreement with the American Can Company. By 1932, Metal Box had cornered the market for tin cans in Britain and, in addition, had agreements with both the leading American concerns, which guaranteed the supply of information on all the latest techniques, machinery, etc. By this time, this one company supplied 90 per cent of all cans to the fruit and vegetable canning industry, and its output rose steadily from 23 million cans in 1930, to over 100 million by 1932.[21] With prices falling after 1931, when a price maintenance agreement in the tinplate industry came to an end, the can supply problem of only a few years earlier, had been virtually eradicated.

Finance

During the twenties the infant canning industry in Britain suffered from a shortage of capital needed to finance the expansion of canning operations. At this time canners usually obtained funds from within a small circle of friends, and by the ploughing-back of profits. By 1930, however, the pressure of demand for British canned produce was so great that access to outside funds became vital if the industry were to be able to expand to meet this demand. A major factor preventing heavy outside investment in the industry at this stage was the element of uncertainty which was associated with canning operations in this country. This was due mainly to the instability of raw material suppliers and to the dominant position held by importers of canned foods in the wholesale and retail markets. Banks were, in general, loath to finance canning operations to any great extent — an important fact since many firms had not as yet sufficient liquid assets to be entirely free of bank finance. Being unfamiliar with the conduct of the business of canning, they tended to apply their usual rules to the calling in of advances after the turn of the year, a practice which had the unfortunate effect of compelling many canners to realise their stock in early spring, often at a heavy loss.

The flotation of the National Canning Company Ltd., in 1931, with a share capital of £350,000 by British Shareholders Trust Ltd., marks the beginning of interest in the canning industry by financiers with capital to spare. From this time on, money poured into the canning industry. The results, however, were not all beneficial. In the words of one observer, 'the advancement of the new industry fell out of the hands of those who could be safely trusted to take a nurse's care of its child, and frustrate any attempt to run before it could walk, into the hands of financiers and capitalists who saw a ready outlet for surplus capital with a profitable return.'[22] Many small concerns sprang up subject to no control, and without the market strength to pursue a rational sales policy. Individualistic policies led to over-production, undercutting, stock-dumping, etc., all of which had serious repercussions on the development of the market for British canned goods, and on the progress of the industry as a whole. Under these circumstances many companies had a struggle to meet dividends during the thirties. In 1934 for example, two of the leading concerns United Canners Ltd., and Beaulahs Ltd., recorded no dividend, and the National Canning Company Ltd., one of the most successful, paid only 5 per cent to its ordinary shareholders. The chairman of Foster Clark Ltd., a leading provisions company which had taken up canning, had to report in 1935 that the canning side of the firm's activities was as yet making no contribution to profits.[25] By the late thirties there was general agreement in financial circles concerning the poor performance of the canning industry. In the words of one commentator: 'Commercially, the industry has been a disappointment. After their early rise during the worst of the depression to almost 50s., the shares of National Canning have been below £1. The new companies have quite failed to make the progress which their directors sincerely forecast at the time of their flotation.'[26]

It seems, perhaps, paradoxical that an over-abundance of capital entering the industry after 1931 should have presented so many problems to canners, when one reflects on the acute shortage of finance before 1930. Clearly, the problem lay not in the excess itself but rather in the effective utilisation of this inflow of capital. In theory, an equitable distribution of incoming finance between the various branches of the industry should have enabled a balanced expansion. In practice, however, the inflow of capital took the form of investment in factories and machinery only. This had the effect of making the industry 'top-heavy', since the means of disposing of the increased output of the rapidly-expanded manufacturing sector were simply not available. The glaring fact was that the market for British canned goods was still in its infancy, and was unable to absorb the rapidly increasing production. Capital was needed for advertisement, for the improvement of marketing facilities, for the co-ordination of raw material supplies, and for scientific agricultural production of an adequate acreage of produce, grown specifically for canning. The fact that capital was not put to the most effective use was due, in great measure, to difficulties in the field of organisation.

Organisation and Marketing

The formation of the National Food Canning Council in 1926 was intended to provide the canning industry with the means of co-ordinating the activities of the various associated interests. Before very long, however, it became blatantly obvious that this body, despite the energetic work of the chairman, Sir Edgar Jones, was no more than a glorified public relations outfit. With progress coming fast in the late twenties, the main activities of the NFCC came to be centred around the promotion of the industry by means of vigorous press campaigns, and the Annual Canners' Convention. While profits were rising and technical difficulties were being steadily ironed out, the need for a strong national organisation seemed superfluous. However, when difficulties in marketing and strain on raw material supplies began to lead to over-production, undercutting, and stock-dumping, the need for a controlling body became increasingly urgent. The formation of the Fruit and Vegetable Canners Association of the United Kingdom in 1931 seemed to provide the answer. At first it provided the necessary debating ground for organisational and marketing problems, and made available the machinery for effective organisation. Unfortunately this body failed to bridge the gap between discussion and effective action. Petty rivalries and lack of cooperation prevented it from playing an effective role during the troubled thirties. So, in the absence of a strong controlling voice in the industry capable of coordinating the activities of canners, the development of a national sales policy which would ensure fair trading methods and the effective channelling of incoming capital was seriously hampered.

It was, in fact, in the field of marketing that the most serious problems existed for the canning industry. The panic dumping of products, persistent over-production, and cutthroat competition led many contemporaries to suggest that by the mid-thirties the market for British canned produce had reached saturation point. This seems hardly credible when one reflects on the fact that, in 1930, consumption of canned food as a whole was less than 4d. per head per week of the population and that of canned fruit and vegetables was only ½d.[27] However, this view is to a certain extent justified, if one considers, for example, canned fish and canned fruits. Clearly, serious problems existed in these branches of the industry, stemming from the very nature of the specific products and the correspondingly entrenched consumer preference for the more exotic imported varieties. In a situation where, for much of the population, the thirties saw a rise in purchasing power, canned herrings, the chief product of the British fish canning industry, had little hope of gaining much of the popularity of canned salmon. Similarly the long-standing popularity of imported canned pineapples, peaches, apricots, etc., presented the canners of British fruits with serious demand problems. To attempt to measure the intractability of these problems however, would require a detailed investigation of the nature of demand for canned produce, which is beyond the scope of this discussion. But the extent of these problems were most certainly accentuated by the lack of cooperation between canners. The success of British canners depended to a great extent upon their ability to penetrate the wholesale market. This was no easy task, even under the most favourable circumstances. Over a period of fifty years, an organisation had been built up by foreign importers through wholesale merchants and retailers in Britain, with all the trade conditions and credit arrangements. Cooperation at national level on such subjects as the planning of output, national publicity, the standardisation of packs, the stabilisation of prices, etc., was essential if a market for British canned products was to be forged successfully.

The condensed milk industry is the exception which proves the point. The establishment of the Milk Marketing Board in 1932, and the subsequent rationalisation of the condensed milk trade, accompanied by restrictions on imports, set the scene for a dramatic increase in the home production of condensed milk. By 1935, over 62 per cent of the 4,451,000 cwts. of condensed milk consumed in the United Kingdom was home-produced, compared with only 26 per cent in 1930.[28] By 1937, the United Kingdom output of condensed and evaporated milk was nearly 4 million cwts., making her the second largest world producer.[29]

In contrast, disorganisation and lack of cooperation were the outstanding features of the fruit and vegetable canning industry during the thirties. Nowhere was this so obvious as in the supply of raw materials. Clearly the availability of constant and adequate supplies was a crucial factor in the field of distribution, if gains were to be made from importers. During the thirties, however, this was never achieved in the fruit and vegetable canning industry, the reason being the failure to stabilise the relationship between canners and the growers of raw materials. This failure led to uncertainty concerning the availability of adequate supplies of fruit and vegetables of the right quality, and in turn to render prices of the finished products liable to wide fluctuation, depending on whether crops were good or bad. The problems in the canner-grower relationship stemmed from two sources. On the one hand, the supply of good quality fruit and vegetables in sufficient quantities for the canning industry's requirements depended to a large extent on the size of the relevant crop but more importantly, on the relative prices farmers could expect from other sources, i.e. the fresh fruit and vegetable markets and jam manufacturers. The fact that British canners were often in direct competition with these other outlets presented serious difficulties, particularly if crops were poor in which case there would be severe competition between canners for available supplies. This was in complete contrast to the American industry, where growers were organised and produced crops expressly for canning. The question of quality was also important in this respect, in so far as the availability of several outlets for their produce did not encourage growers to take much care to plant varieties of fruits and vegetables suited to canning. As a result of this, canners were often forced to take a certain amount of substandard produce rather than face the possibility of being left without any supplies.

On the other hand, many inexperienced canners, rather than commit themselves to long contracts, based on prices which would allow the grower a fair margin of profit, preferred to speculate on a fall in price in the event of heavy crops. More often than not, this either led to panic buying at exorbitant prices in the event of a poor crop, or, in the event of a glut, to serious loss for the grower. Undoubtedly, the inability of canners and growers to establish sound relationships, based on mutual interest by means of long contracts, was an important factor retarding the development of the market for British canned produce. In general, though, the industry was characterised by individualistic policies and unwillingness to enter into agreements. Some of the larger firms were the principal offenders in this respect. With household brand names and established footholds in the wholesale market, they were loath to take part in schemes which might compromise their market position.

The price-cutting, over-production, dumping, etc., which were so common in the thirties reflected the frustration of the many small concerns, who found it difficult to penetrate the wholesale market dominated by the big-name companies. Attempts were made to overcome these difficulties through joint effort. The most notable was the formation of English Produce Canners Ltd., in 1934, by a group of small canners who felt handicapped individually by the lack of capital with which to advertise, and so enjoy the privileges and terms which larger concerns were able to obtain. The scheme brought a number of small concerns under an umbrella selling organisation, using the label of 'English Produce Canners'. Resources were pooled, and each canner was given a quota using the EPC label. Once this quota was filled he could then pack the rest of his produce under his own name. Despite the success of this scheme, other canners were slow to follow the example, and by the end of the inter-war period, little progress had been made towards the kind of rationalisation which had had such a dramatic impact on the condensed milk industry.

The Role of Government

During the twenties, the influence of the government acting through the Ministry of Agriculture and Fisheries was quite important. It was the initiative of some officials at the Ministry which had led to the meeting of 1926, and it was the government which financed Camden and other research institutions. Once the industry began to get off the ground, the government continued to play an active role in smoothing out early difficulties. In 1930, for example, the application of the National Mark Scheme to various English canned products, was intended to boost the prestige of home-produced canned produce. This scheme, under the auspices of the Agricultural Produce (Grading and Marking) Act, was organised by the Ministry of Agriculture and Fisheries in consultation with the National Farmers' Union, the National Food Canning Council, and the wholesale and retail distributive trades. It was intended by progressive standardisation, both of the product and methods of canning, to improve the quality of British canned foods, and thereby to increase their consumption. The scheme was voluntary and indeed, some large canners preferred to remain aloof from it. Nevertheless, a sufficient number of canners entered to make the National Mark label carry some weight. At the close of 1931, of the 59 factories canning fruit and vegetables in England and Wales, 38 were registered packers under the National Mark[30] and by the end of 1933, these figures had risen to 74 and 54, respectively.[31]

How important the application of the National Mark was in stimulating demand for British canned produce is difficult to assess. Contemporaries, at least, were in no doubt. According to one observer: 'the growth of the canning industry is being assisted by the association of the greater part of the industry with the National Mark Scheme. The Scheme is shaping the development of the industry along sound lines with a firm basis in standardised high quality. It has proved a definite selling force'.[32] Most certainly in terms of production, the National Mark played an important role in establishing standards of quality in the industry. Whether it was a 'strong selling force' is a matter of conjecture.

During the thirties, with the exception of the Milk Marketing Board's reorganisation of the condensed milk trade, government activity in relation to the canning industry centred solely around the imposition of duties on foreign canned produce. It was hoped that the duties would give a fillip to sales of home produce. The most significant effect, however, was to increase the share of Empire producers in imports at the expense of foreign producers. Only in the case of condensed milk and canned vegetables did the duty stimulate demand for British produce although imports of canned vegetables continued to increase rapidly. In the case of canned fish, canned fruits and canned meat, no substitution took place; the duty was obviously insufficient to produce a shift in consumer preference away from imported varieties of these products, and as can be seen from Table II, imports of canned fruit and fish continued to increase rapidly in spite of the duty.

Table II: *Retained Imports of Canned Foodstuffs to the United Kingdom 1930-35 (000 Cwts.)*

	1930	*1935*
Meat	1377*	1302*
Fish	1296	1410
Vegetables	751	1287
Fruit	2782	4687
Condensed Milk	2596	1784

Source: Census of Population 1930, 1935.
* includes meat extract. For 1930 – 85,000 cwts. For 1935 – 54,000 cwts.

Even the increase in output of British canned vegetables is less than might have been expected, considering the fact that the home produce was in direct competition with imported canned vegetables. In view of the relative ineffectiveness of the duties and the obvious success of the milk marketing scheme, one is left wondering what might have resulted from similar government action in other branches of the canning industry.

In the final analysis, the performance of the British canning industry during the inter-war years reflected the problems of a new industry attempting to gain a foothold in a market already dominated by established and popular imported products. Progress, it is true, was made, especially in the field of condensed milk and canned vegetables, but the true measure of the achievement of British canners must be the fact that by 1938, Britain still imported five-sevenths of her requirements of canned food and in so doing remained the world's largest importer.

Notes

1. Imperial Economic Committee, *Supplies of Canned and Dried Fruit 1938*, London, 1939, p.7.
2. ibid, *Canned and Dried Fruit Supplies in 1933*, July 1943, p.12.
3. ibid, *Cattle and Beef Survey*, June 1934, p.189.
4. Final report on the 4th Census of Production 1930, Vol. III, p.86.
5. ibid, p.116.
6. ibid, p.86.
7. ibid, p.116.
8. Empire Marketing Board, *Canned and Dried Fruit Supplies in 1931*, EMB, 55, July 1932, p.8.
9. Imperial Economic Committee, *Canned and Dried Fruit Supplies in 1933*, p.7.
10. Empire Marketing Board, op. cit., p.11.
11. Imperial Economic Committee, *Canned and Dried Fruit Supplies in 1934*, July 1935, p.12.
12. Empire Marketing Board, op. cit., p.7.
13. The Annual Report of the Fruit and Vegetable Preservation Research Station, Chipping Camden, Gloucestershire, 1930-31, p.12.
14. ibid, 1932-33, p.17.
15. ibid, 1932-33, p.11.
16. *The Canning Industry*, Vol. II, 1932, p.111.
17. *Food Manufacture*, Vol. IV, 1929, p.72. See also A. Plummer, *New British Industries in the Twentieth Century*, p.231.
18. W.E. Minchinton, *The British Tinplate Industry*, 1957, p.152.
19. ibid, p.190.
20. There were, in fact, several Americans on the board of the British Can Company.
21. *The Canning Industry*, Vol. II, 1932, p.129.
22. *Food Manufacture*, Vol. XIII, 1938, p.206.
23. Imperial Economic Committee, *Supplies of Canned and Dried Fruit 1935*, 1936, p.13.
24. ibid, *Supplies of Canned and Dried Fruit, 1936*, 1937, p.13.
25. *The Economist*, Vol. CXX (29 June 1935), p.1492.
26. *The Canning Industry*, Vol. V, 1935, p.157.
27. *Food Manufacture*, Vol. VIII, 1933, p.223.
28. *The Economist*, Vol. CXXXI (2 July 1938), p.5.
29. O. and T.W. Jones, *Canning Practice and Control*, 1941, p.4.
30. Empire Marketing Board, op. cit., p.8.
31. Imperial Economic Committee, *Canned and Dried Fruit Supplies in 1933*, p.7.
32. *The Canning Industry*, Vol. I, 1931, p.5.
33. Jones and Jones, op. cit., p.2.

PART THREE: A NUTRITIONAL EVALUATION

15 DEVELOPMENTS LEADING TO PRESENT-DAY NUTRITIONAL KNOWLEDGE

DOROTHY F. HOLLINGSWORTH

Lavoisier is usually considered to be the founder of the modern science of nutrition. Just before the French Revolution he and the physicist Laplace demonstrated that there is a relationship between the heat produced by an animal and the respiratory exchange of oxygen and carbon dioxide. They did this by placing a guinea-pig in a small closed chamber surrounded by ice. They measured the amount of ice melted during 10 hours and at the same time the amount of carbon dioxide expired by the animal. Lavoisier also measured the oxygen consumption of men and showed that it increased after food and exercise. He also showed that the nitrogen in the air is not changed during respiration. He communicated his findings in a letter dated 19 November 1790 to Joseph Black, the discoverer of carbon dioxide, who was at that time Professor of Chemistry and Medicine at Edinburgh. During the next century many scientists designed calorimeters in which men and laboratory animals could live for hours or days whilst their metabolism was studied. Among the famous names of the time were Rubner in Berlin, Pettenkofer and Voit in Munich and the great American nutritional scientist Atwater, who was a pupil of Voit. Atwater worked around the turn of the century at Storrs, Connecticut, and he did the experiments which established the essential quantitative physiological knowledge on which all assessments of the energy needs of men are based. Another pioneer in energy metabolism, Benedict, worked with Atwater. Not only did Atwater study energy metabolism: he also showed how to calculate the energy value of diets.

During the nineteenth century the science of chemistry progressed. Early in the century attempts were made to classify foods according to their chemical properties and the French physiologist François Magendie experimented on feeding dogs exclusively on one or other type of food. He showed, for example, that those he fed on fresh meat lived in good health but others, to which he gave only sugar or starch or fat, lost weight and became ill. These and other experiments led him to conclude that foods containing nitrogen are essential for health. Magendie's work was the foundation on which the great German chemist Liebig built. The German work began to attract attention in England in about 1840, but a sensation was caused when two years later Lyon Playfair, who had studied with Liebig at Giessen and who returned to England fired with missionary zeal for his teacher's revolutionary ideas, communicated a short report outlining new theories of the functions of foods to the members of the Section of

Chemistry at a meeting of the British Association for the Advancement of Science at Glasgow. Shortly afterwards the English translation of Liebig's work appeared giving a full account of his theories. He constructed his main theory on the differentiation Magendie had made between nitrogenous and non-nitrogenous foods. The former he regarded as flesh-formers and the latter as the chief source of animal heat and energy, because they contain carbon, hydrogen and oxygen and are oxidised to carbon dioxide and water. One of his classifications of foods was as follows:

| *Plastic Elements of Nutrition* | *Respiratory Elements of Nutrition* |
(Nitrogenous)	(Non-nitrogenous)
Vegetable fibrine	Fat
Vegetable albumen	Starch
Vegetable casein	Gum
Animal flesh	Cane sugar
Animal blood	Grape sugar
	Milk sugar
	Pectin
	Wine, beer and spirits

These views prompted the first scientific and quantitative studies of English diets, which were based on estimations of the amounts of carbon and nitrogen in different foods. The former was regarded as a measure of energy or heat-producing value and the latter as an indication of blood-forming and, therefore, tissue-forming power. The estimates of Edward Smith for the nutritional value of diets and for nutritional needs were made in terms of grains of carbon and of nitrogen.

Liebig analysed a number of his nitrogenous materials and concluded that they all contained the same proportions of carbon and nitrogen. This finding, and other similarities, led him to the erroneous conclusion later known to have resulted from the necessarily crude methods of analysis, that they were identical in composition. A Dutch chemist, Mulder, had reached the same conclusion in 1837 from his analyses of nitrogenous materials. He thought that there was one complex, nitrogen-containing component of all living matter, both plant and animal, and he called it *proteine* (Greek — I take first place). Liebig believed from the results of his chemical analyses that the proteins of milk, eggs, meat and other animal foods, with the one exception of gelatin, were identical in composition with the proteins of plants and he taught that herbivorous animals build up their tissues directly from the proteins of plant foods, being first converted into blood proteins and subsequently into those of muscles and other organs. This simple theory dominated opinions on nutrition for nearly fifty years. Gelatin was an anomaly: it contained nitrogen and yet would not support growth and health, as demonstrated in experiments on dogs and man by Magendie. Liebig looked back on his analytical results and found that there is slightly more nitrogen and less carbon in gelatin than in fibrin or albumen and suggested that it was not an ordinary blood or flesh forming protein. The true explanation was not found until fairly recent times.

Towards the end of the century the orthodox teaching on man's need for food was that there were five *proximate principles* of foods. Three, proteins, fats and carbohydrates, were organic and two, salts and water were inorganic. The proteins were nitrogenous compounds which served, after digestion, to supply material from which the growing animal formed new tissues or the adult replaced 'wear and tear'. They could also serve to supply energy by oxidation if they were not used for tissue-building. The carbohydrates and fats were mainly of use as sources of energy, but could also be desposited in the body as adipose tissue. The mineral salts were calcium and phosphate, used for hardening bones and teeth, sodium and chlorides needed for the blood, iron to form red blood pigment, iodine for the functioning of the thyroid, and also potassium and magnesium. Some authorities added 'accessories' such as condiments, alcohol and caffeine, which might influence nutrition by promoting the appetite or stimulating the body in some other way. Vitamins were nearly discovered in 1881. It was a logical deduction from the theory about protein, fat, carbohydrate, salts and water, that an appropriate mixture of these should provide everything necessary for life. Indeed, Voit suggested earlier that appropriate experiments should be done using pure protein, fat, sugar, starch and minerals constituents – he seems to have suspected that there are other essential substances in natural foods. He rejected the idea of doing such experiments on the grounds that any such food mixture would be so tasteless that no animal, much less man, would eat it.

The problem was eventually tackled along the lines Voit had suggested, but with a different object. Professor Bunge of Basle was interested in the functions in the body of various mineral salts derived from foods. He encouraged a young Russian assistant, Lunin, to try to rear mice on food mixtures which had been so purified that they contained only small residual traces of mineral salts. He found they did not survive long. Next he added various salts and observed that although the mice lived longer they did not thrive. Finally, he added the whole of the mineral ash of milk, thinking that by doing so he would supply all the necessary minerals, but the results were no better. This was unexpected because he had taken great trouble to compound his mixture of purified protein, fat and carbohydrate to correspond to the composition of milk itself. He fed control animals on milk and they flourished. In translation, Bunge wrote:

> It is a noteworthy fact, although animals can live on milk alone, yet if all the constituents of milk which according to the present teaching of physiology are necessary for the maintenance of the organism are mixed together, the animals rapidly die. Cannot cane sugar take the place of sugar of milk? Or are the inorganic constituents of milk chemically combined and only assimilable in this combination? . . . Or does milk contain, in addition to protein, fat, carbohydrates, other organic substances, which are also indispensable to the maintenance of life? . . . It would be worthwhile to continue the experiment.

Unfortunately, Bunge and Lunin did not do this. About twenty-five years later, by almost identical experiments, Pekelharing (in Holland), Stepp (in Germany) and Gowland Hopkins (in England) independently got evidence of the existence of a new class of dietary essential. At about the same time (1907) two Norwegian scientists, Holst and Frölich showed that guinea-pigs developed scurvy if fed the type of foods (deficient in fresh produce) then given to the Norwegian navy. Just before the end of the nineteenth century Eijkman and Grijns in the Dutch East Indies observed that the polishings of rice cured the neuritic symptoms in children fed on a diet of polished rice. Thus it seemed that the polishings contained some dietary essential.

Such dietary essentials were at first called 'accessory factors of the diet' or 'accessory food factors' (cf. Committee upon Accessory Food Factors (Vitamins) of the Medical Research Council). Funk in 1912 coined the name 'vitamine', relating it, in the first instance, to the deficiency diseases beri-beri (lack of vitamin B_1 or thiamine) and scurvy (lack of vitamin C or ascorbic acid) and possibly pellagra (lack of nicotinic acid) and rickets (lack of vitamin D). He thought the substances were 'amines'. In 1920 Drummond suggested the name 'vitamin' to avoid confusion with amines, stating that the name would be acceptable under the standard scheme of nomenclature adopted by the Chemical Society, which permitted a neutral substance of undefined composition to bear a name ending in 'in'.

After the discovery of vitamins, scientific interest shifted from the old proximate principles to this new field. In passing it is interesting to note that the 1914-18 War broke out before the importance of vitamins was fully recognised, but Britain was fortunate in that late in 1916 a committee of physiologists appointed by the Royal Society to advise on physiological matters relating to the war drew up in a confidential document the first estimate of the food resources and requirements of the United Kingdom, and this was later published as *The Food Supply of the United Kingdom* (Cd.8421) HMSO, 1917. This committee, bearing in mind work then current on the cause of beri-beri and scurvy, warned the government that there would be risk if imports of fresh fruit were stopped, as was proposed, that the health of the people would be harmed as a result of lack of 'essential subtle principles'. The government in due course accepted the advice of this committee and managed the food supply for the remaining years of the war according to known scientific principles, with the result that Britain ended the war in better nutritional shape than Germany. Between the wars nutritional interest centred on identifying and synthesising individual vitamins, determining their functions and starting to assess human needs for them in quantitative terms. In 1940, a swing-back began. The limited food supply of many people in Western Europe led to a practical interest in the quantities of food necessary for individuals and for whole populations. British food policy was based on the concept that, provided bread was of good nutritional value and ample supplies of vegetables were available, the nutritional well-being of adults would be maintained if energy needs were met and the determination of energy needs became important. For growing children it was understood that protein and calcium were specially needed and the various milk and other schemes were introduced or extended.

With the growth of the world food problem since the end of the war, entirely new attention has been paid to the protein needs of the very young and to the nutritional properties of different proteins. These depend on the composition of proteins in terms of constituent amino acids and on their digestibility. More recently the relationships between energy and protein have come to be more fully understood and it is now common knowledge that it is wasteful to meet protein needs if energy needs are not fully met. With energy shortage protein is used for the production of energy rather than for growth and development. This concept is discussed fully in *Energy and Protein Requirements,* the report of a joint FAO/WHO *Ad Hoc* Expert Committee.

With the growth of affluence in the western world and the consequent dangers of overnutrition, attention has concentrated on the problems of obesity and the possibility that the diseases of affluence, particularly coronary heart disease and diabetes, may be of dietary origin. This has led to intensive research on the individual constituents of fats and on their metabolic effects and, more recently, on the different carbohydrates and on the indigestible or 'fibrous' parts of foods. Thus, about half a century after it was learnt that proteins, carbohydrates and fats do not form the whole nutritional picture, it is becoming understood that these major constituents of diet may play a much more complex role in metabolism than was formerly believed. Nutritional considerations are now also becoming increasingly complex in other directions. It is known that individuals vary greatly in their needs for energy and for all nutrients, but it is not known why. Thus, estimates of the nutritional requirements of groups of people usually include large safety factors to allow for individual variations. Another complicating fact is the relationships between the various nutrients. It has become recognised that the nature of the diet as a whole can have a major influence on the availability to man of many nutrients. Thus, as already stated, the practical protein value of a diet cannot be considered without regard to its energy value. Or again, many dietary factors influence the amount of iron absorbed from a mixture of foods. Certain vitamins (e.g. nicotinic acid) occur in some natural foods in combination with other organic constituents which render them unavailable, or less readily available to man, without appropriate forms of cooking or other treatment. Thiamine is necessary for the metabolism of carbohydrate. Thus, the more carbohydrate eaten, the greater the requirement of thiamine. One of the amino acids, tryptophan, is a precursor of nicotinic acid (or niacin). Thus, the greater the consumption of tryptophan the lower the requirement of nicotinic acid (it is now usual to combine these two effects by expressing requirements in terms of 'nicotinic acid equivalents').

In recent years there has been a general unease in Britain about the state of both research and communication in human nutrition. One result of this was the appointment late in 1970 of the Joint ARC/MRC Committee on Food and Nutrition Research to advise the Agricultural Research Council and the Medical Research Council on research in food and nutrition and its promotion. The Committee sat under the Chairmanship of Professor A. Neuberger. Its report to the two Councils was published at the end of 1974 'as a basis for discussion both within the Councils and in the wider scientific community, preparatory to the consideration of policy'. Many gaps in knowledge about human nutrition are identified in the report and detailed suggestions for further work are made. The multi-disciplinary nature of nutrition is stressed and three important and urgent areas for research are regarded to be of equal importance: the maintenance of the safety and quality of our food supplies; the role of nutrition in diseases of complex or uncertain aetiology, and the extension of our knowledge of the metabolism of nutrients in order to understand better the nutritional aspects of problems relating to man's future health.

Notes

ARC/MRC Committee (1974), *Food and Nutrition Research,* London, Her Majesty's Stationery Office and Amsterdam – New York, Elsevier Scientific Publishing Company.

Aykroyd, W.R. (1967), *Sweet Malefactor: Sugar, Slavery and Human Society,* London, Heinemann.

Barker, T.C., Oddy, D.J. and Yudkin, John (1970), *The Dietary Surveys of Dr. Edward Smith 1862-3,* London, Staples Press.

Burnett, John (1966), *Plenty and Want: A Social History of Diet in England from 1815 to the Present Day,* London, Thomas Nelson. Published in Pelican Books 1968.

Drummond, J.C. and Wilbraham, Anne (1939), *The Englishman's Food: A History of Five Centuries of English Diet,* Revised Dorothy Hollingsworth 1958, London, Jonathan Cape.

Goldblith, S.A. and Joslyn, M.A. (1964), *Milestones in Nutrition,* Westport, Connecticut, The Avi Publishing Company, Inc.

Joint FAO/WHO *Ad Hoc* Expert Committee (1973), *Energy and Protein Requirements.* FAO Nutrition Meetings Report Series No. 52. World Health Organization Technical Report Series No. 522.

McCarrison, R. and Sinclair, H.M. (1953), *Nutrition and Health,* London, Faber and Faber.

McCollum, E.V. (1957), *A History of Nutrition,* Boston, Houghton Mifflin Company.

McKenzie, J.C. (1965), *The Composition and Nutritional Value of Diets in Manchester and Dukinfield in 1841,* Transactions of the Lancashire and Cheshire Antiquarian Society, Vol. 72 for 1962.

Orr, John Boyd (1936), *Food, Health and Income,* London, Macmillan.

Salaman, Redcliffe N. (1949), *The History and Social Influence of the Potato,* Cambridge, The University Press.

Stewart, C.P. and Guthrie, D. (eds.) (1953), *Lind's Treatise on Scurvy,* Edinburgh, The University Press.

16 SOME BASIC PRINCIPLES OF NUTRITION

JOHN YUDKIN

All living organisms, whether animal or vegetable, need materials that build up their tissues while they are growing, and that constantly make good the wear and tear of these tissues throughout their lives. In addition, they need some source of energy in order to carry out these processes. Green plants get their building materials from the carbon dioxide in the air and from the soil, and their energy comes from sunshine. Animals, including man, get both their building materials and their energy from their food.

We can get a reasonably good idea of how this happens by comparing the human body to a motor car. A very special motor car, it is true, because in its first years it grows from something like a Mini into something like a Rolls Royce. And if all goes well, it keeps itself in good condition for three score years and ten, with reasonably new tyres, constantly charged battery, excellent engine, rust-free body. For this to happen, you need two different sorts of supplies constantly available. You need all the components to keep every part of the motor car in tip-top condition, so that everything is in order and in good repair all the time. In addition, you need a source of energy both for the car to be able to run, and also to do the work of building up the car, during its growth from a Mini to a Rolls, and of restoring the continuous wear and tear on its chassis and body.

Of course no car can itself do this, but this is the sort of thing that the human body can do. Each of the foods we eat almost always contains a mixture of fuel and building components. We can separate these various constituents during the process of digestion, so that when they are absorbed into the body, they circulate in the blood stream to the various tissues in the body that make use of them. The ability to separate food components for our use is, then, one important way in which our bodies are more sophisticated than our motor car. Another way in which we differ from even the most elaborate motor car is in our ability actively to manufacture a great number of the many components our body needs from a much smaller number of building materials. It is as if you were able to provide the car with a mixture of a few metals like iron and chromium and aluminium, together with some silica and a few other materials, and you then found that the car was able to make from these a wide variety of car components such as cylinder blocks, air filters, door handles, tyres, wheels and lots more.

The fact is that the body consists of several thousands of different substances. But it can make almost all of these from a large and unspecific range of other substances. There is only a small number of these that it cannot make, and it is these that make up the *essential* building materials, or nutrients — perhaps forty or fifty of the thousands of substances that go to make our living bodies. These few essential nutrients have to be supplied to the body as such, otherwise it will not be able to continue in health, and indeed may die. The nutrients come to us in our food, together with the sources of fuel or energy. The constituents of our food can be divided into six classes. These are carboyhydrate, fat, protein, mineral elements, vitamins and water.

Water is an essential part of living tissue. Since we are losing water all the time, in the urine, from the skin, in the breath and in the stools, it has to be replenished all the time. We need at least two pints every day, more — sometimes much more — if we are in a hot environment, and especially if in such an environment we are doing a great deal of physical work. We can live for many weeks without food; we can live for only a few days without water. Normally, of course, we do not have to worry; thirst is usually a good indication that the body needs more water. This, however, is less efficient when we suddenly find ourselves in extremely hot and exhausting conditions, where we have to take water even if we are not obviously thirsty.

Apart from water, the body requires materials to be used as fuel, and as replenishment for wear and tear and for necessary growth. These functions are performed by the solid constituents of food. It is usual to say that some of these are used as fuel only, some as nutrients only, while some are used as nutrients or as fuel. We often say that the carbohydrates in our food — the starches and the sugars — are used entirely as fuel. The fat in our food is used largely as fuel, but some particular constituents of fat are nutrients. The proteins in our food are used primarily as a source of nutrients, giving the body its essential amino acids. But the proteins not used in this way are used as fuel. Finally, the mineral elements and the vitamins are entirely used as nutrients. We shall have to modify this simple concept about the strictly fuel functions, or the strictly nutrient functions, of carbohydrate, fat and protein, but we can leave this for a little while.

We can now look more closely at the energy (fuel) and the nutrients supplied by our food. The energy content of food is often referred to as its calorie content. Since energy can be measured not only as heat (calories) but in lots of other ways such as electricity, there is now just one unit used by the scientists for all these forms of energy. This is called the joule. However, I am using calories here since most people will understand this term more readily.

There are two things about energy or calories that are often misunderstood. In the first place, food does not really contain calories in the same way as it might for example contain fat or vitamin C. You can extract the fat or the vitamin C from foods and put these into bottles, but you cannot extract calories and see them. Calories represent the energy that the food can produce when it is used as fuel in the body. In just the same way, you can if you wish talk of the calories in your petrol or the lead in your petrol, but whilst you can extract the lead, you cannot extract the calories. Until the petrol is being used to run your engine, the calories in it represent only the potential energy that can be released in your engine.

The second point worth making is that the word 'energy' as used in nutrition does not have the same meaning as 'energy' used in ordinary day-to-day conversation. When the advertisements say that biscuits give you energy, you should not think that you eat a biscuit and this then enables you promptly to rush out to mow the lawn, or tear round the block on your bicycle. It means no more than saying that petrol gives your car energy. Your car will not go any better by simply adding another gallon of petrol to what you already have in your tank. So to say that food gives you calories or energy is only to say that it is a source of fuel ready to produce energy when you 'burn' it in the body.

Since all foods contain some carbohydrates or fat or protein, or a mixture of these, all foods provide energy. The chief carbohydrates are starch and sugar. Starch is found in potatoes, bread and all cereals. Sugar is found not only in your sugar bowl, but put by the manufacturers into sweets, cakes, biscuits, soft drinks, ice cream and a host of other foods. Lactose is a special sort of sugar found in milk. Small quantities of other sugars in our diet come from fruit and vegetables. The most obvious sources of fat are butter, margarine, cooking oils and fats, and the visible fat in meat. But even lean meat contains a fair amount of fat, and similar 'invisible' fat is found in larger or smaller amounts in milk, fish and even bread. About half of our daily fat comes in these invisible forms.

We always think of protein in terms of milk, meat, fish, poultry and eggs and cheese. Certainly these foods supply a great deal of the protein we consume. But we are wrong if we think firstly that they contain only protein, and secondly that we get no protein from other foods. As we saw, meat and fish, especially fish like herrings, salmon and mackerel, contain quite significant amounts of fat as well as protein, and like most 'solid' foods, quite a lot of water. Secondly, nearly half the protein in our diets comes from other foods. Bread, for example, contains about 8 per cent of protein! Because of the amount we eat, we get on average more protein from bread than we get from eggs and fish and cheese together. This shows how important it is to consider not only how much nutrient there is in an ounce of food, but how many ounces we are eating.

You will remember that what we get out of proteins is the amino acids. We then use these to build up the particular proteins we need in the body. Because of this, some of the proteins in our food are better than others, because they contain a better assortment of amino acids than do other food proteins. On the whole, most proteins from animal foods are better in this respect than are the proteins from vegetable foods. But in practice it doesn't really matter, because we eat so many different foods. As a consequence, what one protein may lack in the way of amino acids is very likely to be made up of a different assortment of amino acids from those in another protein. It is very rare indeed, at least in well-off countries like ours, for anyone to be short of protein. We get much more than the 1 or 1½ ounces that we need each day.

I want now to come back to some dietary items being entirely for energy, some entirely for supplying nutrients, and some for both. It is more accurate to say that *most* of the carbohydrate and fat are used directly for energy, and *most* of the protein indirectly for energy. You will understand what I mean if you follow what happens to any one of these; let us take carbohydrate as an example. At a given moment there are very many — perhaps thousands — of different substances in the body derived from the two or three simple sugars that enter the bloodstream after the digested carbohydrates are absorbed. Some of these derived substances are simply intermediate materials produced as the sugars go through the complex series of chemical changes by which they are burned (metabolised). Some on the other hand appear to be essential for the proper functioning of the body cells and tissues. And some are possibly transitory intermediates, and yet it seems that the body needs them in a fairly constant concentration at all times, even though they are continually being produced and destroyed. Examples of some of the materials I have in mind are cholesterol, citric acid and glyceraldehyde. In fact, all the substances in the body are really only transitory, whether they are there because they have been supplied as such by the diet, or whether they are being manufactured all the time from other dietary materials; there is no tissue in the body, not even the bones, that is not constantly being 'worn out' and reconstituted.

This background gives us a better understanding of the role played by such dietary items as vitamins, and tells us why, for example, protein is used for building body tissues and yet is used as fuel. As to the first, it is important to realise that the body's enormously complex chemical processes involve large numbers of chemical substances. Some of these you cannot make, and so you have to take them in your food; these are the essential nutrients. The others, the greater majority, you can make from a very few basic raw materials in your food, such as carbohydrate or fat. Thus, if anything goes wrong with any of the processes for manufacturing one or more of these very many substances, the consequences could be as serious as is the absence of one of the essential nutrients, such as a mineral or a vitamin, from your food. I shall have more to say about this later on.

We can now unscramble the muddle many of us get into when we are told that protein is used to provide the amino acids to build the body's tissues, and at the same time that all the protein is burned to give calories. What we can now see is that the wear and tear of the body's tissues releases amino acids that were supplied earlier by dietary protein and are now being replaced, and that both these released amino acids and those left over after replacing them are being burned to give calories. Thus, the total quantity being burned is in fact equal to all the protein that you have been eating.

We can now look at the mineral elements and vitamins — what they do and where you find them. All of them are needed in very much smaller quantities than is protein. A day's supply of one of them is at most one-thousandth of an ounce; of others, one ten-millionth of an ounce or less is all that we need for a day. Several of the vitamins and minerals are found in very many foods in more than adequate amounts, so that though they are essential, you are highly unlikely ever to be short. I am thinking of sodium, potassium and phosphorus amongst the mineral elements, and pantothenic acid and pyridoxin and vitamin E amongst the vitamins.

However there are minerals that might be short in our food. The most important are calcium, iron and iodine. Calcium has lots of functions in the body; the best known is that it is needed to build up the bones and the teeth. It is found in largest amounts in milk and cheese; it is also in the soft bones that you might eat in sardines or whitebait for example. Iron is chiefly used in making the colouring matter of the red blood cells. If there is not enough in the diet, the effect is to produce anaemia. The best foods for iron are meat and eggs. Iron is probably the nutrient most likely to be deficient in our lives, especially in women. We need mention only one more mineral element, iodine. In some parts of the world, especially in mountainous areas, this was often lacking in the diet, apparently because it is washed out of the soil. The effect is to produce a swelling of the thyroid gland in the neck, called a goitre, and in children it can lead to cretinism, a disease in which there is a failure to grow physically and mentally. This sort of goitre, however, is much less common now. Partly this is because some countries deliberately put iodine into their salt. Partly it is because improved transport brings iodine-rich foods, such as fish, to what were remote areas.

The vitamins are very different one from the other, and have quite different jobs to perform. It is usual to call them by the letters of the alphabet, since when they were first discovered their chemical composition was unknown. Nutritionists nowadays give them their chemical names when they are known, but most people still use the letters. They are best discussed by seeing what happens when one does not have enough of any one of them. Thus, if there is a lack of vitamin A, one will be unable to see well in the dark. Vision in the light will at first be unaffected, but eventually the eyes will get red and inflamed, and in due course they become so affected as to lead to permanent blindness. But this only happens in severe and prolonged deficiency; nevertheless, it does unfortunately happen in a number of the poor countries of the world. Vitamin A is found in milk, butter, margarine and cheese. Especially rich sources are cod liver oil and particularly halibut liver oil. In addition, it is possible to make vitamin A from a particular yellow material called carotene found in carrots and green leaves and some fruit.

Vitamin D is concerned with helping the body to absorb the calcium from food and to use it for making the bones and teeth. Growing infants especially need vitamin D to protect them from rickets. Adults require very little, if at all. The amounts needed from food will depend on whether or not the skin has access to reasonable amounts of sunlight. This will result in the production of the vitamin in the skin. Vitamin D exists in only a few foods. Milk and butter and margarine contain small amounts, and fish liver oils contain much larger amounts.

In the early days, a vitamin B was described which was needed to prevent beri-beri, a disease found especially in people who eat a lot of polished rice and little else. We now know that the foods that protect against beri-beri, especially liver and the germ of cereals, contain other vitamins, so vitamin B was divided later into vitamin B_1, vitamin B_2 and so on. The other name for vitamin B_1 is thiamine. Mild deficiency leads to weakness, constipation and perhaps slight paralysis, but more severe deficiency produces fully-fledged beri-beri. Of the other vitamins of the B group, we need mention only niacin (or nicotinic acid) and riboflavin. Insufficient niacin leads ultimately to pellagra; insufficient riboflavin leads to sore eyes and inflamed skin, especially of the face and groin. All the B vitamins tend to be found in similar foods. Although rich sources are liver and cereal germ, the inclusion of meat and milk in the diet will ensure adequate amounts; vegetarians will get enough if they include milk or cheese.

One more vitamin, vitamin C, should be mentioned. This is found in fruit and vegetables, and classically scurvy was the result of diets lacking in these foods, especially on long sea voyages. It is easily lost when fruit and vegetables are sun-dried, and quite a lot can be lost by overcooking vegetables and by using excessive amounts of water. Frozen fruits and vegetables, and several sorts of tinned fruits and vegetables can still contain quite a lot of vitamin C. There is some argument as to whether a low intake, but not little enough to produce scurvy, nevertheless leads to undesirable effects. There is also some argument as to whether very large doses of vitamin C can produce good effects, such as immunity to colds. I myself am very sceptical.

17 NUTRITION SURVEYS

D. S. MILLER

Much of this book is concerned with the inter-relationship between the consumer and his diet, and the effect that this has on health. This is a subject that is of considerable importance in the world today since by present estimates about half the world's population is undernourished and many of the remainder suffer from diseases of civilisation associated with the consumption of too much food. The historian might think that with modern techniques these problems could be easily assessed, but there are many difficulties which are similar to those he experiences in making historical assessments. For instance, a competent field worker in rural Africa seldom has sophisticated scientific techniques at hand, and the sort of information that he can collect may often be poorer than that gleaned from parish records in medieval England. There are many reasons for this, but the most important is the illiteracy of the population and hence the absence of written records on basic parameters such as food production, trade, morbidity and mortality. Other difficulties are the logistics and costs of mounting a survey in a country with poor road communications where workers require not only supplies of scientific equipment but also food and some homely comforts to ease life in an isolated environment. It is not surprising therefore that the amount of useful data from many developing countries is sparse and sometimes even non-existent.

Thus the present-day nutritionist dealing with the Third World has to grapple with information which is similar to that available to historians interested in British development over the past two or three centuries. Interestingly, the nature of the societies studied also have some remarkable similarities. In the developing world today one can observe the transition from a rural economy where most of the population are involved in agriculture to an industrial society with its concentration of people in vast conurbations. Cities like Calcutta, Ibadan, and Buenos Aires will be larger than New York, London and Tokyo by the end of this century. In this sense historians interested in the industrial revolution have now in different countries in the world a cross-section in time for comparative study. A village in imperial Ethiopia had much in common with a fifteenth-century English village, certainly in so far as way of life and nutritional status was concerned. And the motivation for peasants to leave their 'green and pleasant land' in developing countries to enter the 'dark satanic mills' must also have much in common with that in England of the eighteenth and nineteenth centuries.

Another similarity of particular interest to the nutritionist is between our diets in history and those eaten in developing countries today, not of course in the actual foods consumed, but in their nutrient content. Thus energy and protein intakes are minimal in both situations, and vitamin and mineral deficiencies are common. These factors and the lack of public health engineering (water supplies and sewers in particular) lead in both to high mortality rates which are compensated for by high birth rates. Thus one finds an increasing population in the midst of chronic undernutrition and occasional famine. The lack of development and hence lack of individual wealth reveals an inability to cushion the worst effects of natural disasters such as drought, pestilence and plague. The Irish potato famine has thus relevance to the famines of today, as has the increased stature of the European population to the stunted growth of children in developing countries, or the high age of menarche in European girls during the last century to present-day population studies. There are however still many gaps in our knowledge. For instance, measles is a killing disease in Africa today, but we do not know if this was the case in Europe in the past. Also we do not know whether low food intakes are due to low food supplies *per se*, an inability to produce more food, or simply that the diets consumed were so monotonous, bulky and unpalatable that appetite was inhibited.

It is apparent therefore that historical studies of countries with developed economies have much relevance to those interested in promoting human welfare in the rest of the world. Whereas one must not be overwhelmed by similarities in development, indications of possible successful courses of action may be surmised. However, it does not follow that all countries will or should follow the same path to Utopia. Nor is it certain that we have moved towards Utopia ourselves. Nevertheless the historian can provide the nutritionist with valuable information and it is appropriate that he is aware of the requirements of the nutritionist and the sort of techniques he currently uses to obtain his data.

Survey Techniques

In most parts of the world nutritional surveys amount to no more than a limited assessment of the food consumed, together with a clinical examination for overt signs of malnutrition. This state of affairs is not so serious as at first appears because impaired nutritional status in the developing countries is often gross and seldom requires subtle techniques for its detection. However, it is important to realise that much of the published information is approximate and is likely to remain so until more funds and more personnel are available for the work. Jelliffe (1966) lists ten sources of information useful for the assessment of nutritional status (Table I). This outline presents a formidable task seldom achieved even in developed countries.

Table I: *Assessment of nutritional status**

Sources of information	Nature of information obtained	Nutritional implications
(1) Agricultural data Food balance sheets	Gross estimates of agricultural production Agricultural methods Soil fertility Predominance of cash crops Overproduction of staples Food imports and exports	Approximate availability of food supplies to a population
(2) Socio-economic data information on marketing, distribution and storage	Purchasing power Distribution and storage of foodstuffs	Unequal distribution of available foods between the socio-economic groups in the community and within the family
(3) Food consumption patterns Cultural-anthropological data	Lack of knowledge, erroneous beliefs and prejudices, indifference	
(4) Dietary surveys	Food consumption Distribution within the family	Low, excessive or unbalanced nutrient intake
(5) Special studies on foods	Biological value of diets Presence of interfering factors (e.g. goitrogens) Effects of food processing	Special problems related to nutrient utilisation
(6) Vital and health statistics	Morbidity and mortality data	Extent of risk to community Identification of high-risk groups
(7) Anthropometric studies	Physical development	Effect of nutrition on physical development
(8) Clinical nutritional surveys	Physical signs	Deviation from health due to malnutrition
(9) Biochemical studies	Levels of nutrients, metabolites and other components of body tissues and fluids	Nutrient supplies in the body Impairment of biochemical function
(10) Additional medical information	Prevalent disease patterns, including infections and infestations	Interrelationships of state of nutrition and disease

*Adapted by Jelliffe (1966) from WHO Expert Committee on Medical Assessment of Nutritional Status.

The first half of Table I is directly concerned with the evaluation of diets. A gross estimate of the availability of food in most countries can be obtained from the annual publication of *The State of Food and Agriculture* (FAO, 1966), which presents the balance of food production, imports and exports in terms of food supplies per head. Such information could be regarded as a 'meaningless mean' since it takes no account of the distribution of food by social and economic class, cultural or anthropological group, or by season of the year. But it does provide a valid comparison from year to year and indicates what might be achieved if it were possible to provide an optimum distribution of food along physiological lines. To measure the extent to which this is achieved it is necessary to complete time-consuming dietary surveys together with extensive laboratory tests.

The second half of Table I is concerned with the measurement of the effects of diets on the performance of individuals. Information on births and deaths is of use in evaluating nutritional status and can be collected by relatively unskilled labour, but the assessment of the prevalent disease patterns, particularly those such as infections and infestations that often lead to or are aggravated by malnutrition, requires skilled diagnosis. A similar skill is also required for the recognition of the physical signs of malnutrition, about which even the experts do not always agree. Probably the most objective measurements are anthropometric and biochemical but, as with the dietary surveys, these are both expensive and time-consuming. Also, one should not have a false sense of accuracy about even these measurements since their validity depends upon the standards against which they are judged. Physiological norms cover a range of values far greater than the precision of the techniques used to measure individuals.

Food Intakes

The assessment of any diet involves measurement of the consumption of food, the conversion of these values into nutrient intakes, and the comparison of these against standards for requirements. Stated simply in these terms, the procedure looks extremely easy, but in fact there are difficulties at every stage. In particular, it is difficult to measure the food intake of individuals since Heisenberg's 'principle of uncertainty', that you cannot measure anything without altering it, applies as much to dietary surveys as to atomic physics and, inevitably, patterns of food consumption change because measurements are being made. This is particularly true in measuring the food consumption of people in the developing countries, and probably the most reliable method, if the most laborious, is to reside with a group of people for long periods of time such that you are regarded as one of them (Culwick, 1951). This procedure also has the added advantage that variations in the consumption of food from day to day, from festival to festival and from season to season, are taken into account. In practice, however, extensive measurements of this type are extremely rare, particularly in the developing countries where the number of trained nutritionists is limited. Most investigators are faced with a choice between studying a small group of families in depth or larger numbers more superficially. The decision will depend upon the objectives of the survey, but in view of the possibility of obtaining gross dietary information from other sources the method of choice is one that gives individual food intakes.

Table II: *Dietary survey techniques*

(1) Measurements as eaten:
    By (a) Direct weighing
          (b) Standard household measures
          (c) Description of portion

(2) Estimations by recall, either from the immediate past (e.g. 24 h recall), or as the usual intake (i.e. 'customary diet'):
    From (a) Description of portions of food
           (b) Frequency of eating the foods
           (c) Standard measures of key foods, e.g. bottles of milk, loaves of bread

(3) Estimations from consumption of groups, e.g. households, villages, regions:
    From (a) Larder inventories and household purchases
           (b) Family budgets and other socio-economic data
           (c) Food production and marketing information
           (d) National production, import and export of food

The various techniques of dietary survey are shown in Table II. Method 1(a) provides the most accurate record that can be obtained, and is the most desirable if one is interested in the distribution of nutrients within a family, or indeed in the dietary intake of individuals. The recommendations for the International Biological Programme give a minimum of 3 days weighed intake of individuals at least twice a year from statistically selected households, but preceded by social (i.e. patterns of food intake) and economic (i.e. food availability) surveys to ensure the validity of the times chosen for measurement. However, the method is expensive of time and skilled personnel, and the investigator may be obliged to compromise some degree of accuracy, in which case diet histories may be obtained either by questionnaire or interview using one of the methods in (2). These techniques must be carefully validated on small samples before widespread use. Alternatively, an estimate may be obtained by a study of food moving into consumption using one of the methods in (3) but, as pointed out above, care must be used in interpreting such surveys since they give no indication of the distribution of food within the group.

Direct weighing is the most accurate, but causes the most disturbance. The use of standard household measures, e.g. cups, spoons, cigarette tins, is reasonably accurate, but estimates based on the descriptions of portions are notoriously inaccurate even when made by skilled personnel. Some studies indicate that the amounts of foods consumed correlate well with the frequency with which they are eaten, but the method needs verification, particularly for any given social setting. Similarly, it has been shown that the intake of some nutrients may be estimated from a knowledge of the consumption of a few specific foods, e.g. calcium intake in Britain may be estimated from the consumption of loaves of bread and bottles of milk.

Nutrient Intakes and Requirements

People eat foods, not nutrients, but it is the nutrients that are important in the assessment of diets. Research relating to nutrition during the past hundred years has demonstrated the need for some 40-50 chemical substances (amino acids, vitamins, minerals, fats, carbohydrates) to be present in an adequate diet. They are required by the body in daily amounts varying from mere traces to several grams, and the need for them has been shown by the remarkable alleviation of clinical symptoms when the pure substance is given, e.g. vitamin B_1 (thiamine) in beri-beri, and vitamin C (ascorbic acid) in scurvy. There is no doubt that the most accurate way of determining nutrient content is to analyse a duplicate portion of everything eaten, and these standards were employed in the survey of diets in British hospitals (Platt, Eddy & Pellett, 1963). In this way not only can the more stable major nutrients be determined, but also the more labile vitamins in samples as eaten. In developing countries, variations between different samples of the same food make this principle more important, but the technique is impractical in most cases. Analysis of similar foods, prepared in a similar way, is possible, but most workers use food tables, which many groups now have on computer tapes and punched cards.

The difficulties associated with the two stages of the assessment of diets can be overcome if there is a sufficiently large team of enthusiasts, but the statement of requirements involves difficulties of a different sort. It frequently surprises people of other disciplines that nutritionists are unable to state with precision an individual's requirement of a particular nutrient. The problems are complex, and national and international committees are set up at frequent intervals to reappraise research and revise the scales. These committees usually state requirements in terms of 'recommended allowances' rather than in terms of a minimum intake. In doing this they provide a safety margin to allow for variations between individuals. They also warn of the dangers of applying their recommended allowances in assessing or prescribing diets for groups of individuals when the distribution of the nutrients within the group is not known. This warning needs to be heeded particularly when considering family intakes since frequently the head of the family, whose nutrient requirements are least exacting, gets the major share of the nutrients. An examination of tables of nutrient requirements as given by different sources shows a range of values larger than can be scientifically justified and which result at best from differences in the way they are intended to be used, and at worst from political interference. For example, the adult human requirement for protein ranges from 40g/day as given by FAO to 140g/day as given by the USSR: similarly the American vitamin C requirement is twice that for other countries. Inevitably, the controversy is often reduced to semantics. Thus 'minimum physiological requirement' (usually reduced to nutrient requirement) is not the same as 'recommended daily intake' (usually reduced to 'nutrient allowance'). For example, it might be possible to get by with a miserable diet containing only 40 grams per day of protein, but one would hardly like to recommend that people should do so.

There is also debate about the meaning of minimal physiological requirements. Should these represent the intake necessary to eliminate overt signs of deficiency or one to provide optimal nutrition? Also should the adopted values be the lowest ever recorded or the average for all measurements? (Yudkin, 1968.) The present trend is for committees to base their figures statistically to cover 97 per cent (i.e. mean + 2 SD) of the population, and such standards can be used to judge the adequacy of individual diets.

Such considerations do not, nor can they, take into account that the requirements for several nutrients are affected by the rest of the diet. Thus the ratio of protein:fat:carbohydrate affects the requirements of riboflavine and thiamine, and the requirements of vitamin D and calcium are dependent on the amount of phytate in the diet. Nor do accepted requirements allow for man's ability to adapt to undernutrition in its many forms, and one should not automatically expect classical signs of deficiency disease simply because survey results indicate that the intakes of many individuals are chronically sub-optimum.

In view of these problems some workers prefer an 'appeal to the rat' in assessing diets, and will conduct elaborate feeding trials using laboratory animals to settle the finer points of evaluation, but the cost of such experiments is normally prohibitive. Nevertheless it is appropriate to assess the diet as a whole following an examination of each separate nutrient, if only on paper.

Energy

The primary value of a diet is determined by its energy content, since if this is not adequate to meet requirements for maintenance, activity, and in the case of children growth, all dietary constituents will be used in an attempt to meet energy requirements and will not be available for other more specialised purposes. Workers in Ceylon (Baptist and de Mel, 1955) have shown that the growth rate of young children, 1 – 6 years old, eating an entirely vegetable diet with an adequate caloric intake was greater than that of those eating a mixed diet (i.e. containing animal protein) which was deficient in calories. Elaborate and detailed investigations as to the nutrient content of the latter diet are not relevant since the limiting feature of the diet is its energy content. Man's need for fuel is paramount. Lack of calories presents the most important nutritional problem in the world today and the chief symptom is loss of weight or failure to grow properly. In extreme cases one has the picture presented by the Oxfam posters. Other symptoms are lassitude and lowered work rate in the adult population, with considerable social and economic repercussions. The tendency in western societies is for both calorie intakes and average weights to be slowly increasing, and clinicians are becoming concerned about the increasing prevalence of obesity and associated degenerative diseases. Thus, whilst energy foods are a necessary condition to being energetic, eating them does not necessarily provide *joie de vivre,* and an excessive consumption frequently has the reverse effect.

Protein

Protein is not only a source of calories, but is also required for growth and maintenance of the tissues. Approximately one-tenth of man's diet should be protein, which is conveniently that proportion found in most staple foods. There are however three important exceptions, i.e. cassava, sago and plantain, and it is mostly in areas where these foods are consumed that young children suffer from kwashiorkor. The dual function of protein is further complicated by the differences in protein quality, which are dependent upon its amino acid composition. For instance, whereas egg protein may be completely utilised for body building, a protein such as gelatin would be entirely rejected because it lacks one of the essential amino acids – tryptophan. In between these two extremes lie other foods and, generally speaking, animal proteins are superior to those from plant sources, although there is a considerable overlap. However, quality ratings of this sort are not meaningful because people do not eat single sources of proteins and when several sources of protein are consumed together there is a supplementary effect between the amino acid pattern of each. In this way, two proteins of low biological value can yield a mixture of high value because the deficiencies of one can be made up by the excesses in the other. By eating a varied diet and protein from a wide range of sources it is possible to make 2 + 2 = 5, an apparent trick which is very useful. Because of this we state requirements in terms of an 'ideal' protein — Net-dietary protein: actual protein requirement will be greater depending upon the quality of the diet.* Although adults require more protein each day than their children, the required percentage in their diet is more or less the same because they eat so much more food. Apart from the newborn, most individuals could satisfy their need by eating bread alone.

However, it must be pointed out that these calculations do not hold if the calorie intake is low, since under these conditions protein will be preferentially burnt for energy purposes. Because of this complication, nutritionists nowadays do not distinguish between protein deficiency and energy deficiency but refer to protein-energy malnutrition (PEM) which covers the broad spectrum of symptoms from kwashiorkor to marasmus to hunger oedema. Children just do not eat enough of diets low in protein, and are thus concomitantly deficient in calories: similarly, those eating diets low in calories are forced to burn what protein there is for energy purposes. The evaluation of diets indicates that the primary cause of protein malnutrition is insufficient food, although the secondary causes may range from failure of breast-feeding to a gastro-intestinal infection. Two corollaries follow from this reasoning. Firstly, if simple calorie deficiency does not exist, then the addition of empty calories in the form of sucrose or fat to the diet is unwarranted, and secondly if simple protein deficiency does not exist, the value of protein-rich foods have been overrated. What is required is enough of a balanced diet, which is of course the panacea for all nutritional problems.

Minerals

About one-hundredth part of the diet consists of essential mineral elements which are primarily involved in skeletal development and water balance. About twelve elements are important; they may be divided into major and trace according to the quantities required. Of the major elements, sodium, potassium and chloride are found universally in all tissues whether of plant or animal origin, and therefore rarely present nutritional problems. Calcium, phosphorus and magnesium are associated with bone growth,

*In order to calculate the net-dietary protein equivalent of any given diet, it is necessary to know the amino acid composition and from this it is possible to calculate a 'protein score'. The steps in the calculation of protein score depend upon finding which of the essential amino acids would limit the synthesis of body protein, and the protein score is then used to predict the efficiency of conversion of dietary protein into body protein. The product of protein consumed and the efficiency of its utilisation gives net-dietary protein.

but of these only calcium is likely to be deficient in diets since it is notoriously low in the cereals and other staple foods. Dietary deficiencies of phosphorus and magnesium are not known to occur in man. In the British diet calcium is not a problem because of our high consumption of milk and the compulsory addition of calcium carbonate to flour. The absorption of calcium is known to be influenced by vitamin D, and some other nutrients. Also, absorption is influenced by phytic acid, a compound common in cereals. McCance and Widdowson (1942) were the first to show with human volunteers that calcium is less freely absorbed from diets consisting largely of brown bread than from those consisting largely of white, and this led the British Government to add calcium carbonate to bread of high extraction during the war. However, more recent evidence suggests the importance of adaptation to diets high in cereals and phytic acid. There can be no question that many people throughout the world succeed in calcifying their teeth and bones while subsisting for long periods on diets of this kind. Similarly, it is known that man can adapt to diets of low calcium intake, and this is supported by observations made in Ceylon, India, Africa and South America. It must be admitted therefore that because of the many factors regulating the absorption and excretion of calcium it is very difficult to express calcium requirements in precise terms.

Iron is the most important of the other minerals. In man, the turnover of iron is only about 1mg/day, but the higher recommended intakes are necessary because of the low absorption of iron from food. A deficiency of iron leads to anaemia, but anaemia is not always due to a poor diet. Menstrual losses of iron put women at greater risk of anaemia than men. In developing countries the most important mineral deficiency is of iodine, which causes goitre and it is estimated that there are 200 million who suffer from this easily preventable disease.

Vitamins

In contrast to the mineral elements, the vitamins constitute only one thousandth part of a normal diet. However, the absence of one of them can cause spectacular deficiency diseases of considerable importance in history. All the vitamins have now been synthesised and can be manufactured very cheaply. Nevertheless deficiencies do still occur in the world. The nomenclature of the vitamins is confusing to the uninitiated because each is known both by a letter given when its effects were first discovered, and by a chemical name given when its structure was elucidated. Whereas direct weighing is the most accurate method for estimating the adequacy of diets, it must be admitted that the technique is not satisfactory for the calculation of vitamin intakes because the vitamin content of foods is so variable. It depends very much on the age and variety of the plant, the season of harvest, the period of storage and the method of cooking. Most workers therefore rely on clinical signs of nutrient deficiencies in people consuming the diet. A description of these symptoms is inappropriate here and the reader is referred to books (Jelliffe, 1966) which give photographs for ease of identification. The most common vitamin deficiency in the world today is that of vitamin A (retinol) which accounts for 100,000 cases per annum of blindness in S.E. Asia alone. In Britain, in the past, deficiencies of vitamin D (calciferol) causing rickets and of vitamin C (ascorbic acid) causing scurvy were most prevalent.

Nutritional Status

Nutritional status may be defined as the extent to which a customary diet meets individual requirements. As explained above the mainstays of the field worker conducting a nturitional survey are the assessment of the food consumed and a search for overt signs of malnutrition. The historian (Barker, Oddy & Yudkin, 1970) can also do both although so far he has concentrated only on the former. Estimates of mortality and morbidity are however also relevant and heights and weights can be deduced from historical evidence. Even vitamin deficiencies may be inferred from the study of skeletons and food availability. An examination of the paintings of old masters can reveal something of the prevalence of rickets and obesity. It is clear that the application of modern nutritional knowledge to historical studies has only just begun, but it promises to be very fruitful not only to academic historians but also to nutritionists concerned with the Third World and hoping to avoid the mistakes of the past. Food consumption in the developing countries is low but the capacity to produce food is improving. If the economic demand rises, there is little doubt that we shall see the development of food industries similar to our own. The problem at the moment is that the economic demand for food does not equal the physiological need. As the standard of living rises we can expect an improvement in nutritional status, but it is not inevitable. Populations can and do dissipate increased wealth on the status symbols of the affluent societies such as bottled beer, Coca-Cola, and confection. This is not so dissimilar to our addiction to gin in the eighteenth century, which also had a disastrous effect on nutritional status;

Conclusion

I have tried to present an appraisal of the present state of knowledge in this field. Whether it is interpreted as indicating that nutrition is an imprecise science or a fascinating but complex multidiscipline depends on one's point of view. However, I hope the outline of the techniques used by nutritionists may prove useful to historians in interpreting their data. There is no doubt of the value of their findings to nutrition.

Notes

Baptist, N.G. and de Mel, B.V. (1955), *British Journal of Nutrition,* 9, p.156.
Barker, T.C., Oddy, D.J. and Yudkin, J. (1970), *The Dietary Surveys of Dr Edward Smith, 1862-3,* Staples Press.
Culwick, G.M. (1951), *Diet in the Gezirs Irrigated Area, Sudan,* Publ. No. 304, Sudan Survey Department, Khartoum.
Jelliffe, D.B. (1966), *Monograph Ser. W.H.O.,* No. 53.
McCance, R.A. and Widdowson, E.M. (1942), *Journal of Physiology,* 101, p.44.
Platt, B.S., Eddy, T.P. and Pellett, P.L. (1963), *Food in Hospitals,* Oxford University Press.
Yudkin, J. (1968), *Science Journal,* 4, p.48.

18 A NUTRITIONAL ANALYSIS OF HISTORICAL EVIDENCE: THE WORKING-CLASS DIET, 1880–1914

D.J. ODDY

By the late nineteenth century, the degree of industrialisation and urbanisation in Britain had already produced marked effects in British society; Henry Pelling has pointed to the homogeneity of experience which had created a working class; the British urban market had brought about the development of food technology to meet its demands. This is not a period in which the basic question was how to get food to the towns, but one in which many businessmen were concerned with problems of how to extend the life of perishable food, how to provide food of a legally-required minimum quality and, even, how to create substitutes for those foods such as dairy produce which remained high in price. The period I have suggested, therefore, is one when urban consumers were already being supplied with roller-milled flour, early forms of margarine and condensed milk, and cheap jams which were notable for their high sugar content.

As far as working-class diet is concerned the risk is that its boring and monotonous nature may not seem a subject likely to interest people: there is none of the glitter of menus and banquets which John Burnett described in *Plenty and Want;* no one in the working class is concerned with the service of meals in French or Russian style. Nevertheless, some historians have brought preconceptions to the study of this period which confuse rather than clarify the issues: Professor W.W. Rostow and Dr. H.L. Beales have both regarded the late nineteenth century as a period of rising food consumption; on the other hand J.C. Drummond thought it a period of widespread malnutrition.[1] Contemporaries were clearly unsure of the position and the question of physical deterioration which arose in the years following the Boer War, while not proven by the evidence considered in the 1904 inquiry, lurked in the back of their minds in view of the inquiry's revelations and the fear of future wars.

If the late nineteenth century was in fact a period of rising living standards then one might assume greater wealth would alter dietary patterns. Drummond expressed this most clearly as

> The decline in the consumption of bread and flour to which we have referred is an interesting phenomenon which began to be evident in Great Britain and the United States late in the nineteenth century ... It seems to be related to a rising standard of living for the falling curve representing bread

and flour is complementary to the rising curve for sugar and sweetmeats. It is also related to a rise in the consumption of meat. These relationships reflect the fact that bread is the staple food of poverty and that people eat much less of it when they can afford to buy meat and to indulge in the type of dish with which sugar is eaten.[2]

To test such a model and, at the same time, the validity of historians' preconceptions of the period, it is necessary firstly to express working-class food consumption in quantitative terms, secondly to make a nutritional analysis of the evidence to provide an objective assessment of its value, and thirdly to evaluate any assessment of the diet through an understanding of the relationship between the diet and epidemiological and social indicators of the well-being of the population. For this purpose, it is possible within the period of this paper, to examine 17 surveys providing a total of nearly 2,500 budgets almost all of which are from working-class families. An analysis of these budgets may go some way to answering the obvious questions about working-class diet: how did they manage? how much did they eat? was it enough?

The Importance of Income

Expenditure on food by working-class families was limited by low incomes. The broad outline is fairly clear: in 1886, almost 25 per cent of adult males earned less than 20 shillings per week, while the wage census of 1906 revealed that

> for the United Kingdom as a whole the weekly rates of wages (exclusive of bonus, if any) of over one-fourth of the adult workmen fell below 20s., and those of nearly two-thirds below 25s., while rather less than a fifth were rated at 30s. or more.

In 1911, an estimate by A.L. Bowley put 32 per cent of the 8 million men regularly employed in the United Kingdom below 25 shillings per week.[3] Low incomes (for the supplementary earnings of wives or children were never large) and irregular employment were normal for many of the unskilled labour employment groups and were reinforced by poor housing and low educational levels. Some indication of these effects in general terms were made by contemporaries: Charles Booth, for example, believed that the lowest income groups, or '"very poor" — are at all times more or less "in want". They are ill-nourished and poorly clad.'[4] While this represented only a small proportion of the working classes the wages paid for unskilled labour in general were, in Rowntree's view 'insufficient to provide food, shelter, and clothing adequate to maintain *a family of moderate size in a state of bare physical efficiency'*, which meant that 'every labourer who has as many as three children must pass through a time, probably lasting for about ten years, when he will be in a state of "primary" poverty; in other words, when he and his family will be underfed.'[5] Booth, however, felt that regular employment was the distinguishing feature in the working class which brought families into the 21 to 30 shillings per week level of income and was 'more than any other, representative of the "way we live now".'[6] Food expenditure was the largest item in family budgets. Nearly 60 per cent of income was spent on food in the surveys carried out before 1900, and generally over 60 per cent was spent in the following decade. Perhaps surprisingly, most money was spent on meat, with the majority of families spending over one-quarter of their food budget on various forms of meat. Even in surveys where the levels of income were especially low, the expenditure on meat remained important; in Rowntree's survey of York, for example, in which roughly half the working-class families examined earned under 21 shillings per week, total meat expenditure was almost one-third on the food budget.

Because of the cost, however, meat and also dairy produce were eaten only in small amounts in these families for whom the staple commodities of the diet remained bread, and, to a lesser extent, potatoes. Thus meat, in Rowntree's words, was often 'a flavouring rather than a substantial course', or, to quote Mrs. Pember Reeves:

> The tiny amounts of tea, dripping, butter, jam, sugar, and greens, may be regarded rather in the light of condiments than of food.[7]

These small amounts, however, were essential to make the semblance of a meal in diets with a high starch content. Charles Booth thought that recognisable meal patterns were found from the unskilled labourer's family (provided he was in regular employment) upwards through the social scale. This meant:

> Meals are more regular. For dinner, meat and vegetables are demanded every day. Bacon, eggs and fish find their place at other times. Puddings and tarts are not uncommon, and bread ceases to be the staff of life. Skill in cookery becomes very important, and though capable of much improvement, it is on the whole not amiss. In this class no one goes short of food.[8]

Booth's experience might have been true for the man of the house, or the lodger, as Booth himself had been, but for the women and children (and probably the whole family when employment was irregular) the struggle to maintain meal patterns was enormous. For example, for midday dinner, potatoes

> are an invariable item. Greens may go, butter may go, meat may diminish almost to vanishing-point, before potatoes are affected. When potatoes do not appear for dinner, their place will be taken by suet pudding, which will mean that there is no gravy or dripping to eat with them. Treacle, or — as the shop round the corner calls it — 'golden syrup', will probably be eaten with the pudding, and the two together will form a midday meal for the mother and children in a working man's family.[9]

This clearly illustrates the complementary nature of certain foods: some form of fat or sugar was an essential component of a meal to accompany the main, and largely starchy, food. In the absence of animal food sugar acted as a substitute and this in turn determined the type of starchy food eaten. Among country families, Rowntree noted other devices to overcome the shortage of animal fats. Even in what he termed 'better-off families' there was

> a good deal of pastry consumed. Some housewives make nearly half the flour into pastry. This might seem an extravagance, but it must be remembered that the pastry is extremely plain and extremely solid. It is usually regarded by the worker as more satisfying than bread; and it saves butter.

The alternative was to make dumplings which used very little lard, suet, or dripping and a very few currants.[10]

Meal patterns within the family are important both in terms of choice of food and the amount consumed. Diets with very low fat content limited the housewife's method of cooking and making meals, quite apart from any restriction imposed by lack of facilities or knowledge. In the towns, perhaps particularly in London, where some areas of large houses had degenerated into multi-occupancy, families frequently lacked cooking facilities which meant that 'the culinary art, if practised at all, is reduced to its crudest form of expression'.[11] Mrs. Pember Reeves, who was an experienced visitor of such homes in south London, agreed that 'In houses where no gas is laid on, the gas-stove cannot take the place of the missing oven, and it is extraordinary how many one-roomed dwellings are without an oven.' Even in the country Rowntree noted that good ovens were exceptional so that bread was seldom home-baked. Newer houses had ovens too small for a large baking and were therefore wasteful of fuel.[12]

Factors of this kind made meal preparation a drudgery and the diet monotonous. Among poor London families Mrs. Reeves concluded: 'The diet where there are several children is obviously chosen for its cheapness, and is of the filling, stodgy kind. There is not enough of of anything but bread. There is no variety. Nothing is considered except money.' At Corsley, Maud Davies noted agricultural labourers' families in which 'the wife cooks only once or twice a week during the winter. She cooks oftener in summer when potatoes are more plentiful.' It was exceptional to find a women who, like 'Mrs T has been a cook and takes pride in her cooking and housekeeping. She cooks every day.' Among the overcrowded London families Mrs. Reeves found no similar example; in her experience 'the Lambeth woman has no joy in cooking for its own sake'.[13]

The eating of food, therefore, was seldom a social occasion. Among Liverpool dock labourers' families:

> The custom of entertaining friends by inviting them to share a meal does not seem much in vogue in homes of this class. Indeed it would appear, perhaps owing to the unattractive character of most of the food consumed, that eating is regarded much less as one of the pleasures of life than among those who pride themselves upon their warm intellectual interests. 'Women wouldn't thank you for a cup of tea,' said one housewife wonderingly, when asked if she never had a friend to tea.[14]

The funeral was a possible exception. In Middlesborough, Lady Bell noted:

> A funeral indeed is one of the principal social opportunities in the class we are describing. 'A slow walk and a cup of tea' it is sometimes called, and the busy preparations in the house for a day or two before, the baking, the cleaning, the turning out, are undoubtedly often tinged with the excitement and anticipation of an entertainer.[15]

Otherwise the normal week's menu showed little variation:

> To boil a neck (of mutton) with pot herbs on Sunday, and make a stew of 'pieces' on Wednesday, often finishes all that has to be done with meat. The intermediate dinners will ring the changes on cold neck, suet pudding, perhaps fried fish or cheap sausages, and rice or potatoes. Breakfast and tea, with the exception of the husband's rashers, consist of tea, and bread spread with butter, jam or margarine.[16]

In Scotland, there was often less variety still in the midday meal when the family were together at home:

> There is very little variety in the dinners provided. Where the mother is at home 'broth' is the staple dish. It is generally made with ½ lb. boiling beef, 1*d*. of leeks, carrots and turnips and ½*d*. barley. The meat is eaten with the potatoes as a second course. If the family are economising ¼ lb. of beef, with 1*d*. bone or parings will be used; and there is no second course.[17]

Meal patterns centred around the presence or absence of the man of the house. When his times of eating differed from those of his children, as they often did, children's meals followed a less regular pattern largely because of the simplicity of their diet:

> Bread, however, is their chief food. It is cheap; they like it; it comes into the house ready cooked; it is always at hand, and needs no plate and spoon. Spread with a scraping of butter, jam, or margarine, according to the length of purse of the mother, they never tire of it as long as they are in their ordinary state of health. They receive it into their hands, and can please themselves as to where and how they eat it. It makes the sole article in the menu for two meals a day. Dinner may consist of anything from the joint on Sunday to boiled rice on Friday. Potatoes will play a great part as a rule, at dinner, but breakfast and tea will be bread.[18]

Among poorer families, the children 'have "pieces" whenever they ask for them' and this was acceptable to mothers if it kept children away from the table while their father ate meat or fish.

Clearly, managing on limited incomes involved a careful distribution of food between different members of the family. There is very little direct evidence to support the general assumption that in the nineteenth century family the father as breadwinner, especially when engaged in manual labour, was entitled to as much food as would satisfy him. Animal food in particular, such as meat and fish, was largely consumed by him for his dinner or as 'relishes' for his supper. The typical nature of this pattern had been observed by Dr. Edward Smith in 1863:

> The meat or the bacon, when the whole quantity is small, as 2 lb. to 4 lb., is commonly cooked for this (Sunday) dinner, and all partake of it. What is left is reserved for the husband, who either takes a little portion with him for his dinner daily, or eats it at home; and it is remarkable that this is not only acquiesced in by the wife, but felt by her to be right, and even

necessary for the maintenance of the family. The remark was constantly made to me, 'that the husband wins the bread, and must have the best food'. If the family be thrifty, the husband will have a morsel of meat or bacon daily throughout the week, but in other instances the whole is consumed in the first two, three or four days. The important practical fact is however well established, that the labourer eats meat and bacon almost daily, whilst his wife and children may eat it but once a week, and that both himself and his household believe that course to be necessary, to enable him to perform his labour.[19]

Charles Booth obviously implied a similar distribution when he wrote 'a good deal of bread is eaten and tea drunk especially by the women and children' and the pattern in London did not change within the following twenty years. Mrs. Reeves found that 'Meat is bought for men, and the chief expenditure is made in preparation for Sunday's dinner, when the man is at home. It is eaten cold by him the next day.' The man also in her estimate, consumed the entire purchase of bacon and half of all the fish bought.[20] The view of one witness before the Committee on Physical Deterioration that 'if the mother does do any cooking it is only for the father', makes more sense when viewed in this light.[21]

Food Supplies

An attempt to quantify what people ate might start with estimates of food supply. Table I shows the United Kingdom food supply for the late nineteenth and early twentieth century expressed as weekly amounts of foodstuffs per head of population, and averaged for the periods 1899-1903 and 1904-1913 to coincide approximately with groups of family budget surveys. Agricultural statistics are better from the mid-eighties onwards and this table is based on the calculation of home production (less seed allowances, or stock of animals, and allowing for industrial consumption) plus retained imports of foodstuffs. This table shows only the principal foods in the diet and, by its nature, conceals some variation in amounts of particular commodities supplied. However, in general terms, there is no reason for supposing that the food supply was unable to keep pace with population growth in this period, but rather that supply was remarkably stable. Few new foods entered the diet within this period and the impact of processed foods such as condensed milk and margarine is often exaggerated, as their use probably was most important within food manufacturing industries or for commercial catering purposes. In fact, the rate of growth of food technology was perhaps the most important factor restricting

Table I: *Weekly* per capita *Food Consumption Based on Supply Estimates*

	Bread (lb.)	Potatoes (lb.)	Sugar (oz.)	Fats (oz.)	Meat (lb.)	Milk (pt.)
1889–1903	6.7	3.2	22.9	21.6	2.2	3.3
1904–1913	6.9	3.6	23.8	22.6	2.2	4.1

the introduction of new forms of food. The technological application of the new science of bacteriology began to affect baking, meat and fish preservation and refrigeration, and dairy produce only from the 1890s onwards. Its effect in the food industries was to introduce standardisation of products, to extend their marketable life and, by shortening curing or ripening processes, to obtain cost reduction. The process was far from complete at the outbreak of war in 1914, although the effect on the consumer had already caused discussion about the disappearance of the traditional diet as an increasing blandness in the flavour of food and less local variation in products was noted.

When expressed in a similar way, family budget evidence for this period shows some clear differences from supply estimates. Table II is based on family budget evidence from the surveys listed in the

Table II: *Weekly Food Consumption of Working-Class Families in Dietary Surveys*

Weighted mean for years:	Bread (lb.)	Potatoes (lb.)	Sugar (oz.)	Fats (oz.)	Meat (lb.)	Milk (pt.)
1887–1901	6.7	1.6	14.4	5.2	1.4	1.4
1902–1913	6.6	3.0	15.5	7.6	1.2	1.8

Appendix. These surveys have been grouped and the figures in Table II are the weighted means per head of the principal items of foodstuffs consumed.

The total number of nearly 2,500 budgets is a large body of evidence, even though it is clear that this cannot be regarded as a sample for the period in statistical terms. Yet there is always the temptation to make sweeping generalisations on the basis of family budget surveys. Lord Boyd Orr succumbed, making his analysis of 1,152 budgets from differing years and sources a basis for generalising about the diet of the whole population. Earlier, Rowntree himself wrote in his conclusion of 'the startling probability that from 25 to 30 per cent of the town populations of the United Kingdom are living in poverty'[22] and following the publication of his book, 6 million hungry people became a political catchphrase. Yet the limitations of this evidence must not be overlooked, since much of the evidence was obtained by questionnaire. Thus most investigations provided a rigid structure which must necessarily have inhibited divergent answers, and insight into consumer behaviour is thus reduced. Also, since there are only the printed versions of these inquiries available as source material, the amount of rounding off and standardising carried out remains unknown.

Despite the variation in sources and methods, the similarity of the results obtained when these diets were analysed suggests that there is some basis for regarding them as normal for working-class families of the period. Although it has been questioned whether London and York provided typical backgrounds from which to generalise,[23] this evidence is from a much wider range of locations. Of the 151 budgets analysed for the period 1887 to 1901, 24 per cent were from the Midlands and industrial North of England, including some from Manchester, Sheffield, West Riding textile towns, Tyneside and Northumberland mining districts. Examples from London, which were not solely those obtained by Booth, accounted for 19 per cent of the total. Towns in England which were primarily non-industrial (and here York was included) formed 16 per cent of the total and a similar proportion came from Scottish towns. In the much larger urban inquiry of 1904, evidence was provided from each region of the United Kingdom, so that between 1902 and 1913 any bias was towards Scottish and Irish urban districts rather than London.

It is also clear that these diets cannot be dismissed as reflecting only the conditions of the 'very poor'. The official inquiries by questionnaire in 1887 and 1904, which obtained their responses through the agency of labour organisations, produced a large proportion of replies from better-off workmen. In the 1904 urban inquiry, for example, 31 per cent of the returns were from workmen whose family income was 40 shillings a week or more, a level attainable in the Edwardian period by only a small minority of the working classes.

In Table II the estimated consumption of bread[24] shows a remarkable similarity to the average figures in Table I. Other estimates in Table I, however, generally exceed the consumption by working-class families shown in Table II.

With regard to potatoes, it should be remembered that several investigators noted the difficulties of obtaining correct consumption figures, particularly when garden produce formed a source of supply. It is possible, therefore, that the figure of 1.6 lbs. potatoes for 1887-1901 is too low to be general among the working classes. The figure for 1901-13 of 3.0 lbs. potatoes seems more in accordance with the estimated consumption of 3.6 lbs. since quite large and somewhat arbitrary allowances were necessary in its calculation. As an estimate, 3.6 lbs. was slightly higher than that calculated by Prest, but just under Salaman's figures.[25]

The difference in sugar consumption between Tables I and II is also due, at least in part, to a methodological point. Table II records sugar consumed in the household in solid form and as treacle or syrup. It therefore omits sugar in manufactured foods consumed outside the home and, although such food expenditure was least in the working classes, budgets showing any sizeable expenditure on food consumed away from home were excluded from the analysis. The estimated total supply of sugar in Table I exceeds household consumption by the amount used industrially (including brewing and food industries). If, in Table I, total supply was deflated by a third to allow for industrial consumption, the remainder or domestic supply would average just under 1 lb. per week, thus comparing closely with sugar consumption in Table II, which may be taken to be almost exclusive of alcohol. In most investigations there was little reference to alcohol, which may therefore be assumed to have been almost entirely consumed outside the home.

The difference in the consumption of animal foods given in Tables I and II cannot be explained in the same way. Although there are considerable difficulties in estimating the production of dairy produce and other fats and little evidence of the industrial consumption of fats, the underlying factor explaining the difference between *per capita* estimates and working-class dietary evidence must be a socio-economic one. Animal foods were expensive relative to vegetable foods, with the differential between them possibly still increasing, as it appears to have done throughout the nineteenth century. As a result, even when a large part of food expenditure went on animal food such as meat, the amounts bought remained small. However, the importance of these items in the diet has already been stressed, and it should be remembered that the monotony of the diet was an important factor in determining total food consumption. If the food available was insufficiently palatable, then it was difficult to eat enough to satisfy the body's needs.[26] The limited consumption of animal foods indicated their use in the working-class diet as a vehicle for consuming larger amounts of carbohydrate foods and it is probable, therefore, that when the animal food content of the diet was reduced by economic factors, the consumption of starchy foods was restricted in turn. Rowntree recorded a family in Essex which, 'though they never felt actually hungry after their dinner, they were never "completely satisfied like", except on Sundays'.[27]

Nutrient Intakes

The food value of the supply estimates (Table I) is expressed in Table III as the daily nutrient value available per head of the population, while in Table IV the nutritional analysis of the family budgets is expressed as the daily nutrient intake per head, averaged out for

Table III: *Daily Nutrient Content of Diet Based on Supply Estimates*

	Energy Value (kcal.)	Protein (g.)	Fat (g.)	Carbo-hydrates (g.)	Iron (mg.)	Calcium (g.)
1889–1903	2,983	73	143	363	11.2	0.47
1904–1913	3,171	77	154	381	11.8	0.54

the periods 1887-1901 and 1902-1913.

The most marked difference between Tables III and IV is the excess of calories and fat in the supply estimates. This can be resolved by examining the difference of 85 grams of fat for 1889-1903 and 89 grams for 1904-13, which, since 1 gram of fat produces 9 calories, explains a difference of some 750–800 calories between the two sets of figures. Intake of other nutrients in these two tables appear to be

Table IV: *Daily Nutrient Intake of Working-Class Families in Dietary Surveys*

Weighted mean for years:	Energy Value (kcal.)	Protein (g.)	Fat (g.)	Carbo-hydrates (g.)	Iron (mg.)	Calcium (g.)
1887–1901	2,099	57	58	336	10.0	0.31
1902–1913	2,398	71	65	375	12.1	0.46

within a similar range so that the *per capita* estimated diet confirms the typicality of the survey evidence apart from the fat content. In this case, it seems that the dietary survey evidence is more valid. If the fat content of the diet was as high as the estimates suggest, then the proportion of calories derived from fat would be 48 per cent of the total. This proportion is even higher than modern British diets in which only 40 per cent of calories are from fat.[28] Before the Second World War about 39 per cent of calories were obtained from fat, while Boyd Orr's figures for 1931-35 suggested that the working-class fat intake provided just under 34 per cent of calories.[29] Thus there are several indications that the proportion of fat in the diet has been rising during this century, and that the lower proportion of fat in the diet suggested by the survey analysis (about 27 per cent) is closer in line with the trend than the higher proportion resulting from the supply estimates.

If Table IV expresses the nutritional value of diets that were probably typical of many working-class families, the next question concerns their adequacy. Intakes expressed per head may seem somewhat unreal in the family context; in some cases such as, for example, a family consisting of a man, a woman and a breast-fed infant it might seem unrealistic to divide the food supply between three persons; but it should be understood that requirements of most nutrients are broadly similar at any age between 7 and 70 years. The conclusion seems inescapable that families in this period with an income of less than, say, 30 shillings per week and with a family of growing children might well obtain only 2,000—2,200 calories and 50—60 grams protein per head per day. Given that the distribution of food within the family followed the general pattern suggested, it is impossible to envisage how the diverse physiological needs of a manual worker, his wife, and growing children could be met adequately. The inference which can be drawn from Smith, Booth, or Rowntree — first-hand observers of the working-class home in the second half of the nineteenth century — is that under these conditions women and children were under-nourished. Rowntree's summary of the situation was:

> We *see* that many a labourer, who has a wife and three or four children, is healthy and a good worker, although he earns only a pound a week. What we *do not* see is that in order to give him enough food, mother and children habitually go short, for the mother knows that all depends upon the wages of her husband.[30]

This distribution pattern of food within the family appeared to be normal behaviour implicit in working-class culture, and it was reinforced by patterns of food choice which were largely limited by social convention and habit. Whether or not the need was for more energy, social emulation required that more meat or dairy produce was bought as income rose. When A.L. Bowley evaluated conditions in towns in 1913, the 'New Standard' he adopted modified Rowntree's diet by including meat, since 'in fact, a workman would sacrifice part of the defined necessaries in favour of a meat diet'.[31] Middle-class advice, therefore, was of little avail: working-class families showed little interest in increasing their intake of vegetable proteins. Dunlop, commenting on the diets of Edinburgh labourers, wrote: 'There is a relatively great use of more expensive foods such as beef, milk, and eggs, and a relatively small use of some cheaper food, such as oatmeal, peas and barley.'

Similarly, he noted that as one penny spent on margarine produced 435 kcals. compared with 1860 kcals when spent on sugar: 'for this reason in the dietaries of the poorer classes the fats should be cut down as much as possible, and the energy should, as far as digestion will allow, be supplied in carbohydrates.'[32] This obsession with the energy-cost of the diet completely ignored the palatability of the foods involved and their acceptability within the family. Although sugar is palatable, starchy foods by themselves are not and it is well-established that energy intakes rise with the proportional increase in fat in the diet. Rowntree noted the implications of middle-class demands for 'economy' by the working classes: 'It means that a wise mother, when she is tempted to buy her children a pennyworth of cheap oranges will devote the penny to flour instead.'[33] It remained for Mrs. Reeves to comment somewhat tartly upon the reality of middle-class advice within the working-class environment:

> There are those who, if they happen to read these weekly menus will criticise with deep feeling the selection of the materials from which they are composed. It is not necessary to pretend that they are the absolute best that could be done, even upon that money. It is quite likely that someone who had strength, wisdom and vitality, who did not live that life in those tiny, crowded rooms, in that lack of light and air, who was not bowed down with worry, but was herself economically independent of the man who earned the money, could lay out his few shillings with a better eye to scientific food value. It is quite as likely, however, that the man who earned the money would entirely refuse the scientific food, and demand his old tasty kippers and meat. It is he who has to be satisfied in the long run, and if he desires pickles, pickles there will be. The fact that there is not enough money to buy good healthy house-room means that appetites are jaded, and that food which would be nutritious and valuable, and would be eaten greedily by people who lived in the open air, seems tasteless and sickly to those who have slept four in a bed in a room 10 feet by 12 feet.[34]

Since the analysis of almost 2,500 budgets of working-class families now suggests that inadequate diets extended further among unskilled workers than merely casual labourers earning a pound a week or less, the question arises of to what extent the effects of inadequate diets were noticeable among the working classes in general. If the families which were investigated were atypical of the working class as a whole, there should be no corroboration from other observers of the effects of poor diet. However, it seems significant that opponents of Booth and Rowntree never offered any contrary evidence on the question of diet. C.S. Loch, for example, perhaps Rowntree's chief critic, concentrated his attack on statistical interpretation rather than budgetary evidence.[35]

Furthermore, Helen Bosanquet's *Social Conditions in Provincial Towns,* while claiming to present a more balanced picture of Britain than could be obtained by relying on evidence from London, included the remarkable sentence: 'Facts and figures are a weariness and for the most part convey little enlightenment.'[36]

In fact, confirmation that the effects of inadequate diet were discernible in Britain can easily be found. In Edinburgh, Paton *et al.* noted that 'in our town there are hundreds of families, the head or heads of which indulge not moderately, but immoderately, in drink.' When family income was reduced in this way, it was not surprising 'that the children are puny, and that the adults are poorly developed and inefficiently equipped for the struggle of existence'.[37] Whether the consumption of alcohol was a cause or effect of poor nutrition was a debatable point among contemporaries. Despite the general view before the Committee on Physical Deterioration that drink caused poverty, other witnesses felt that 'people who have not enough food turn to drink to satisfy their cravings'. Put another way, it seemed that 'The poor often drink to get the effects of a good meal. They mistake the feeling of stimulation after alcohol for the feeling of nutrition.'

The effect of inadequate nutrition on the condition of children was put before the same Committee by a factory inspector, Mr. H.J. Wilson. In textile factories, he explained, for a boy of fourteen

> The hours will be long, fifty-five per week, and the atmosphere he breathes very confined, perchance also dusty. Employment of this character, especially if carried on in high temperatures, rarely fosters growth or development; the stunted child elongates slightly in time, but remains very thin, loses colour, the muscles remain small, especially those of the upper limbs, the legs are inclined to become bowed, more particularly if heavy weights have to be habitually carried, the arch of the foot flatens (sic) and the teeth decay rapidly.

Girls, he added

> exhibit the same shortness of stature, the same miserable development, and they possess the same sallow cheeks and carious teeth. I have also observed that at an age when girls brought up under wholesome conditions usually possess a luxuriant growth of hair, these factory girls have a scanty crop which, when tied back, is simply a wisp or 'rat's tail'.[38]

There are, however, no adequate anthropometric data to confirm such general descriptions of underdevelopment, although some evidence both of the secular trend in physical growth of children and the difference between socio-economic classes does exist.[39]

More specifically, it seems likely that children in particular suffered from the shortage of animal foods in the diet. The excessive part played by cereals and the limited use of dairy produce made rickets exceedingly common among children before 1914, while insufficient animal foods which include readily available iron may have produced conditions of anaemia. The shortage of animal fats was also likely to have contributed to vitamin deficiency in children. But before the concept of vitamins had been developed, what could not be a nutritional deficiency resulted from insufficient food had to be explained as the result of 'improper food', either in terms of choice or quality. This was adopted in the Committee on Physical Deterioration's report which devoted a separate section to improper feeding. The habit of children eating tinned salmon, raw herrings, bloaters, and fried fish among other foods — frequently when fed by parents off their own plates — was deplored, though this was one of the few possible sources of animal food for children who might receive little other than some meat at Sunday dinner.

In some cases, clear signs of vitamin deficiencies were recorded. Dr. Eicholz, reporting to the Committee on Physical Deterioration noted the 'harshness, roughness of the skin' in children with defective nutrition, adding that other characteristics included 'dry, thin, and short or wispy' hair,[40] a phrase echoed by other commentators. In rural areas the analogy was obvious: 'Hard, dry, "staring" hair', wrote a Scottish school medical officer, 'is just as much a sign of defective nutrition in the child as in the animals of the farmyard.'[41]

Nutritional deficiencies were certainly thought by contemporary observers to be factors contributing to the incidence of disease in infancy and early childhood. With over 140,000 deaths of children under 5 years forming almost 28 per cent of all deaths in England and Wales in 1913, Dr. Arthur Newsholme indicated very clearly the importance of the child obtaining an adequate diet to build up resistance to infectious diseases: 'In all these diseases the influence of the previous nutrition of the infant has great importance, and rickets is very commonly the factor in a child's condition which determines the fatal result of any infection by which it is attacked.'[42] As the machinery for medical inspection in schools was fairly complete by 1911, it became clear that 'defective nutrition stands in the forefront as the most important of all physical defects from which school children suffer.'[43] Although medical inspection produced evidence of 'sub-normal' nutrition reaching alarming proportions both in urban and rural areas, the general relationship between nutrition and health in children could not be resolved: 'It is certain that malnutrition and physical defects are closely associated and react upon each other', wrote Dr. George Newman, the Chief Medical Officer to the Board of Education, 'but it is difficult to determine their exact relation in each child, or to say in what degree malnutrition causes other physical evils.'[44]

Dr. Newman's statement highlights the considerable similarity in terms of nutrition and health between Britain in the nineteenth century and developing countries at present. Direct evidence of food consumption in developing countries is also limited and there are major problems involved in adequately assessing the health and nutritional status of any population in aggregate terms. In these conditions, nutrition aid programmes today examine vital statistics with great care for possible indicators of malnutrition amongst the most vulnerable sectors of the community, namely mothers and young children. In Britain, the high infant mortality rates up to the 1914-18 War certainly suggest poor nutrition *and* hygiene, but the pre-school child mortality rate (deaths of children aged 1 to 4 years per 1,000 children in that age group) has been suggested by the

Table V: *Child Mortality Rate in England in the Late Nineteenth Century*

	Child Population (aged 1 – 4 years) (000s)	Deaths in 1 – 4 years (annual averages) (000s)	Child Mortality Rate (per 1,000)
1871–1880	2,576	80	31.2
1881–1890	2,783	75	27.0
1891–1900	2,857	69	24.3
1901–1910	2,991	55	18.4

World Health Organisation[45] as another and possibly more specific indicator of malnutrition if the rate in any population is higher than 10 per thousand. For England and Wales, Table V shows values well in excess of this figure throughout the late nineteenth and early twentieth centuries, and suggests how the use of such indicators designed for developing countries may provide an important perspective of British society in the past. For this period in Britain, some corroborative evidence does exist: but it was not until 1917-18, when the First World War reached its climax, that the medical inspections under the Military Service Acts revealed the extent to which the health of the adult population had been affected by their childhood and upbringing in pre-1914 Britain.

Appendix

The family budgets analysed in this paper are taken from the following sources.

1. *Returns of Expenditure by Working Men*, P.P. 1889 (C.5861), LXXXIV.
2. C. Booth, *Labour and Life of the People*, Vol. 1, 1889.
3. Economic Club, *Family Budgets: being the income and expense of twenty-eight British households 1891–1894*, 1896.
4. T. Oliver, *Lancet* (1895), I, 'The Diet of Toil'.
5. G. Von Schulze-Gaevernitz. *The Cotton Trade in England and on the Continent*, 1895.
6. B.S. Rowntree, *Poverty: A Study of Town Life*, 1901.
7. D.N. Paton, J.C. Dunlop and Elsie Inglis, *On the Dietaries of the Labouring Classes of the City of Edinburgh*, 1901.
8. *Consumption of Food and Cost of Living of Working Classes in the United Kingdom and certain Foreign Countries*, P.P. 1903 (Cd. 1761), LXVII.
9. *Second Report by Mr. Wilson Fox on the Wages, Earnings and Conditions of Employment of Agricultural Labourers in the United Kingdom*, P.P. 1905 (Cd. 2376), XCVII.
10. *Second Series of Memoranda, Statistical Tables and Charts*, P.P. 1905 (Cd.2337), LXXXIV.
11. Dundee Social Union, *Report on Housing and Industrial Conditions*, 1905.
12. Lady Florence Bell, *At the Works: A Study of a Manufacturing Town*, 1907.
13. Maud F. Davies, *Life in an English Village*, 1909.
14. B.S. Rowntree and May Kendall, *How the Labourer Lives: A Study of the Rural Labour Problem*, 1913.
15. D.E. Lindsay, *Report upon a Study of the Diet of the Labouring Classes in the City of Glasgow*, 1913.

Notes

1. H.L. Beales, *Econ. Hist. Rev.*, V (1934), pp.65-75; W.W. Rostow, *British Economy of the Nineteenth Century*, 1948, pp.90-91; J.C. Drummond and Anne Wilbraham, *The Englishman's Food*, 1957 edn., p.403.
2. Drummond, p.299.
3. *Report on an enquiry by the Board of Trade into the Earnings and Hours of Labour of Workpeople of the United Kingdom*, P.P. 1912–13 (Cd.6053), CVIII, xiii. See also P. Snowden, *The Living Wage*, 1912, p.28.
4. *Labour and Life*, I, p.131.
5. Rowntree, *Poverty*, pp.133, 135.
6. *Life and Labour*, V, p.329.
7. Rowntree and Kendall, p.308; Mrs. Magdalen S.P. Reeves, *Round About a Pound a Week*, 1913, p.103.

8. *Labour and Life,* I, p.50.
9. Reeves, p.98.
10. Rowntree and Kendall, pp.39-40.
11. *Report of the Inter-Departmental Committee on Physical Deterioration,* P.P. 1904 (Cd.2175), XXXII.
12. Reeves, p.111; Rowntree and Kendall, p.40.
13. Davies, pp.211, 214; Reeves, pp.103, 112.
14. Liverpool Economic and Statistical Society, *How the Casual Labourer Lives,* 1909, xxiv.
15. Bell, p.119.
16. Reeves, p.111.
17. Dundee Social Union, p.31.
18. Reeves, pp.97-8.
19. *Sixth Report of the Medical Officer of the Privy Council,* P.P. 1864 (C.3416), XXVIII, 249.
20. Reeves, pp.97, 103.
21. *I-D. Ctte. on Phys. Det.,* para.290.
22. *Food Health and Income,* 1936; Rowntree, p.301.
23. W. Ashworth, *An Economic History of England, 1870-1939,* 1960, pp.251-2.
24. All forms of bread and flour consumed are expressed as bread in Tables I and II.
25. A.R. Prest, *Consumers' Expenditure in the United Kingdom, 1900-1919,* 1954, p.51; R.N. Salaman, *The History and Social Influence of the Potato,* 1949, p.613.
26. J. Yudkin, 'Patterns and Trends in Carbohydrate Consumption and their Relation to Disease', *Proc. Nutr. Soc.,* **23**, p.149.
27. Rowntree and Kendall, p.240.
28. See Annual Reports of the National Food Survey Committee.
29. S. Davidson and R. Passmore, *Human Nutrition and Dietetics,* 1969, 4th edn., p.111; see also *Food, Health and Income.*
30. Rowntree, p.135, note 1.
31. *Livelihood and Poverty,* 1915, p.80.
32. Paton, Dunlop and Inglis, pp.87, 73, 9.
33. Rowntree and Kendall, p.312.
34. Reeves, p.131.
35. *I-D. Ctte. on Phys. Det.,* paras.140-141, 161-162.
36. *Social Conditions in Provincial Towns,* 1912; in *The Poverty Line,* 1903, her criticism was limited to a methodological point.
37. Paton, Dunlop and Inglis, p.86.
38. *I-D Ctte. on Phys. Det.,* paras.140-141, 161-162.
39. See J.M. Tanner, *Growth at Adolescence,* 1961, 2nd. edn., Ch. V, especially pp.137-55.
40. *I-D. Ctte. on Phys. Det.,* Q.450.
41. *First Report on the Medical Inspection of School Children in Scotland,* 1913, para.81, cf. Davidson and Passmore, p.489.
42. *Report on Maternal Mortality,* supplement to the *44th Ann. Rept. of the Local Government Board,* P.P. 1914-16 (Cd.8085), XXV, 19.
43. *Ann. Rept. of the Chief Medical Officer to the Board of Education, 1910,* P.P. 1911 (Cd. 5925), XVII, para. 38.
44. ibid., paras. 39, 314.
45. *WHO TECH. REP. SER.,* 1966, No. 340.

INDEX

abbatoirs 49-50, 51, 55
Abernethy, Dr. John 18
advertising 32, 34, 38-40
Aerated Bread Company 164
agricultural labourers 103-16
alcohol consumption 86, 98-9, 140, 144, 162-3, 223, 227; and working class living standards 117-34; brewing 119; changing 124-30; duty on 119, 120, 131; energy value of, in diet 121-4; expenditure on 119-21; prices 119-21, 128-30; regional variations in 119
Aldercroft, D.H. 88
Alexander, D. 156, 158
Allen, David 99
Allied Bakeries 29
Amalgamated Master Dairymen 74
American Cereal Company 35
amino acids 198-200
Anderson, Alexander 33
animals *see* meat industry *and specific types of animal*
artificial insemination 53-4
Association of Biscuit Manufacturers 23-4
Atwater, W.O. 189

Baker Perkins Ltd. 22
bakery industry 29
Bakewell, Robert 47
Beales, H.L. 214
Beck Cereal Company 33
beet sugar 59, 60
Benedict, F.G. 189
biochemistry of meat 54
Biscuit industry 15-27; brands 23; changes in demand for biscuits 24-6; mechanisation of 20-22; production process 16-22
Booth, Charles 120, 122, 123, 215-17, 220
Bosanquet, Helen 226
Bowley, A.L. 225
Boyed Orr, Lord *Food, Health and Income* 73, 221, 224
bread 29-33, 141, 142, 169, 222; demand for 29, 129; prices 106, 107; specialities 30-33
breakfast cereals 33-40; British market for 35-8; consumption of 36-8; marketing 38-40; production of 41
breakfasts 37-8
British Sugar Corporation 63
Brooke Bond Company 96, 170
budgets, family 221-3
Bunge, Prof. 191-2
butchers, 49, 54-5
butter 107

Cadbury Company 79, 81, 83, 84, 88, 89
calcium 200, 210-11
calories 197-8, 208-10, 224; intake of 123, 124
cannibalism 45
canning industry 173-85; American influence on 176-7; finance of 178-80; organisation and marketing 180-83; products 174-5; role of government in 183-4; technology 175-8
capital, industrial 88-9
Captain's biscuit machine 19
carbohydrates 191, 193, 194, 197, 198, 199, 223
carcase meat animals 47-8
Carr and Bagshaw (Sheffield) 154
Carr, John D. 18
Carr & Co. Ltd. 21, 22-3
catering 161-72
cattle 47-8, 54, 55
Cattle, Albert 148
Chambers of Agriculture 74
cheese 107, 144
children 227-8
chocolate 82-4
cocoa industry 77-90; advertising 87; alkali additive 82; changing image of 86-7; consumption 77-9, 81, 85-8; foreign influence on 83-5; imports into Britain 77, 83-4, 87; international trade 83; markets 77, 79; medicinal properties claimed for cocoa 87; prices 78; product variety 80; raw materials 85; structure and

organisation 79, 88; technological innovation in 79-83, 86
coffee 78
coffee public houses 86, 162-3
Coffin, Admiral Sir Isaac 19-20
commodity markets 96
condensed milk 66-7, 181, 184-5
consumer goods 127-9
consumers: expenditure 28; preferences 138-47 *see also specific commodities*
consumption patterns 99-100; changing 124-31
convenience foods 25-6, 34
co-operative societies 70
Co-operative Wholesale Society 23, 156
Corn Law (1815) 158
cost of living 103-16; fluctuations in 106-7
Cracknell machine 19
Crawford, W. & H. Broadley *The People's Food* 135
culture 9

Dance, George 155
Davies, Maud 218
diet: energy values 121, 197-8, 208-9; in history compared with today 2-3, 212; low fat 217; milk consumption 73; patterns 99-100; substitution 106; urban 159; working class 214-31 *see also* food *and* nutrition
dietary change 41
dietetics applied 33
digestion 196
Dodd, George 149
drink *see* alcohol consumption
Drummond, J.C. 192, 214
drunkenness 119, 126

Eastern Counties Dairy Farmers Society 70
Eden, Sir Frederick 141
Eicholz, Dr. 228
English Produce Canners Ltd. 182-3
Evans, Estyn 141
Exall, William 19
Express Dairies 70, 75, 164

family, distribution of food within 219-20, 225
fancy biscuits 17-20
farmers 142; milk trade 65-75 *passim*

fashion 140
fats 191, 193, 197, 199, 224
flour 154; confectionery 29
food: classification of 191; energy content of 197-8, 208-9; importance given to 9; manufacture 169-72; imports 127; supply 220-23; technology 220-21; working class consumption of 214-31 *see also specific foods*
food habits 135-47; highland versus lowland 140-44; North versus South 137-40
Food Machinery (Mather and Platt) Ltd. 177
Foster Clark Ltd. 179
fruit 181-2, 193
Fruit and Vegetable Canners Association 180
Fruit and Vegetable Preservation Research Station 175-6
Fry Company 79, 83, 88, 89
Funk, C. 192

General Mills 39
Gerrard, F. 47
Gilbert, F.W. 70
Graham, Sylvester 31
Grant, Sir Thomas 17, 19
Great Western and Metropolitan Dairies 70
Grocers Federation 24
grocery trade 23, 148-60, 171; customers 149; investment 155; range of goods sold 152-3; specialisation 152

Hilton, G.W. 158
Hobsbawm, E. 125
Hoskins, W.G. 141
Hovis Limited 31-3
Huntley, Thomas 19
Huntley and Palmer 19, 21, 22-3, 25
hygiene 67-9, 72-3; meat industry 52-3, 54

infant mortality 68
iodine 200, 211
iron 200, 211

Jacob's (Dublin) 23
Jefferys, J.B. 152, 156
Jelliffe, D.B. 203-5
Jenson, L.B. 49

233

Jepson, Arthur 163
Joseph Baker and Son 22

Kellogg, Dr. John H. 33
Kellogg, Co. 34, 35, 36, 38

Lancashire 145
Laplace, Pierre S. de 189
Lavoisier, A.L. 189
leather 107
legislation 158
Levi, Leone 119, 120
Liebig, J. von 189-90
Lipton company, Thomas 96, 97-8, 153
Loch, C.S. 226
Lockharts 163
luxury commodities 84, 106, 139-40, 150-51, 154-5
Lyons and Co. Ltd., J. 161-72; Corner Houses 167-8

Macfarlane Lang 23
MacKenzie, W.A. 122-4
McVitie and Price 23
Magendie, François 189
malnutrition 2-3, 205, 214-31 *passim*
Manbre and Garton group 63
mass production 150-51
Mathias, P. 154
Mayhew, H. 162
meals 24-5, 217-20; patterns 217-20
meat industry 44-57; breeding 53-6; consumption 55, 223; eating meat 44-5; meat packing industry 51; prices 106, 107; production 50, 52; refrigeration 50, 51; slaughtering 49-50, 51; trade 48-53
Menier company 80, 84
Metal Box Company Ltd. 177-8
Metropolitan Dairymen's Association 74
microbiology 52, 54
Midlands, the 144-6
milk chocolate 82-3
Milk Control Board 71
Milk Marketing Board 76
milk trade, London 65-76; bottling 67, 75; consumption 67, 73, 144; deliveries 67; government control of 70-71; hygiene 67-9, 72-3; prices 66, 70, 74-5; production costs 71; surplus over liquid consumption 66;
testing 67; transport 75; wholesalers 65, 69, 70, 75
Minchinton, Walter 177
mineral salts 191, 193, 197, 200 210-11
Ministry of Agriculture and Fisheries 174, 183
mobility 138
muesli 40
Mulder, G.J. 190
multiple stores 151, 171

Nabisco company 36
National Association of Biscuit Manufacturers 24
National Canning Company Ltd. 179
National Canning Council 174
National Farmers' Unions 69, 74
National Federation of Dairymen's Associations 74
National Food Canning Council 180, 183
National Food Survey 136, 137, 146
National Mark Scheme 183-4
Newman, George 228-9
Newsholme, Arthur 228
nitrogen 189-91
nutrition: assessment of nutritional status 203-5, 212; analysis 11; basic principles 196-201; knowledge 189-203; measurement of intake 205-7, 223-9; nutrient content of food 207-8; research into 195; standards 117, 123, 124, 131; surveys 202-13

occupations 138
Oliver, Dr. William 18
overnutrition 193, 209

Palmer, George 18-20
parish workhouses 103-4
pasteurisation 67, 69, 72, 75
Paton, D.N. 227
Pearce and Plenty 163, 165
Peek Frean and Company 20, 23, 25
Perky, Henry D. 33
personality 138
pigs 46, 48, 54, 143, 144
Poor Law Unions 104
population growth 55, 98
porridge 38

Post, Charles W. 33, 34
Postum Cereals 35, 38
potatoes 129, 222
poverty 73
Prewett, F.J. 75
prices 103-6
protein 11, 56, 190-91, 193, 197, 198, 208, 209-10
provision dealers 149-50
public health 72-3
Pyke, M. 9, 56

Quaker Oats 35, 36, 38
Quakers 18

Rank Hovis McDougall 30
Reeves, Pember 217-18, 220 226
Rennie, Sir John 17
retailing 148-60
Rostow, W.W. 214
Rowntree, Joseph 119
Rowntree, Seebohm 117, 120, 123, 215-6, 221
Rowntree company 79, 81, 89

sample surveys 135-7
Saul, S.B. 88
Scola, R. 157
Scotland 142-4
Shaw, G. 157
sheep 46-7
Sherwell, Arthur 119
ship's biscuits 15-17
shops 155-8
Shredded Wheat 35, 38
Simmonds, W.H. 153-4
Sims, George 120
Smiles, Samuel 131
Smith, Edward 190
Smith, Richard 31
social class 138
soya bean 56
standard of living: and milk consumption 73; and cocoa consumption 82; in underdeveloped countries 212; of agricultural labourers 103-16; working class 26, 117-34
starch 198
sterilisation (milk) 67, 69
sugar 198; consumption 145, 222-3
sugar trade 58-64, 150, 153, 154; duty on 61; English 59, 62-4; export subsidies 61-2; price trends 62-3, 106, 107;

refining 58-9, 61, 62; technical innovations 60
Sweden 143
sweet foods 145

taboos 9
tallow 107
Tate and Lyle company 63
tea 78, 91-100, 150, 153, 154, 169-70; consumption 91, 92, 99; demand for 98; imports 91, 92; merchanting methods 96; prices 97-8, 99, 107; re-export trade 91; retailing 96-7; technology 96
teashops 164-72
temperance catering 162-3
temperance reform 124,132
Throgmorton restaurant 166-7
tinplate 177-8
tobacco 130
Tooke, T. 149-50
Trocadero restaurant 166
truck shops 158
tuberculin tests 68
Tyneside 144-6

unemployment 107-11
United Dairies 70-71, 72, 74, 75
Ure, Dr. Andrew 22

Van Houten company 80, 81-3, 87
vegetables 181-2
Vicars, T. and T. 21-2
vitamins 11, 191, 192, 194, 197, 200-201, 207, 211-12
Voit, K. von. 191

wages 26; and drink consumption 124-30; purchasing power of 107-8; rise in 117; working class 215-20
Wales 140-41
water 191, 197
Weetabix Ltd. 35, 36
West Country 146
Westerfield, R.B. 156
Whittock, N. 155
wholesaling 148-9
Williams, Stenhouse 72-3
Williamsons, G.H. 177, 178
Wilson, H.J. 227
working class diet 214-31

Zeuner, F.E. 46, 47

235